THE FEEL-GOOD PREGNANCY COOKBOOK

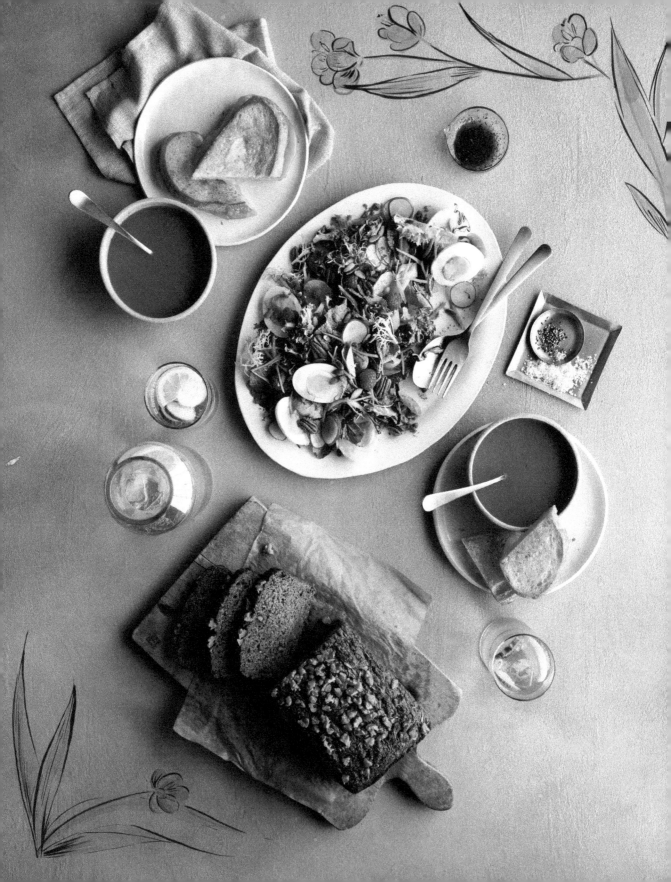

The *Feel-Good* PREGNANCY COOKBOOK

100 Nutritious and Delicious Recipes for a Healthy 9 Months and Beyond

Ryann Kipping, RDN, CLEC

PHOTOGRAPHY BY
Elysa Weitala

ILLUSTRATIONS BY
Vivian Shih

ROCKRIDGE
PRESS

Interior and Cover Designer: Emma Hall
Art Producer: Karen Beard
Editor: Vanessa Ta
Production Manager: Riley Hoffman
Production Editor: Melissa Edeburn

Photography 2019 © Elysa Weitala; food styling by Victoria Woollard, except pp. 3, 21, 36, and 118 © Nadine Greeff.

Illustration ©Vivian Shih.

Author photo courtesy of © Kambria Fischer Photography.

ISBN: Print 978-1-64152-688-3 | eBook 978-1-64152-689-0

R1

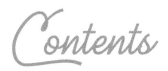

Contents

Introduction IX

Chapter One: FEEL GOOD, PREGNANT 1

Chapter Two: FIGURING OUT WHAT TO EAT 11

Chapter Three: BREAKFAST 27

Blueberry Pecan Pancakes	28
Carrot Cake for Breakfast	29
Cheesy Mini Quiches	30
Chorizo-Potato Hash	31
Egg in Tomato Bake	32
Open-Face Egg Sandwich	33
Egg, Bacon, and Veggie Breakfast Bake	34
Scrambled Egg Pita Pocket	35
Protein-Packed Strawberry Smoothie	37
Mango Carrot Smoothie	38
Veggie-Filled Omelet	39
Kiwi, Cucumber, Kale Smoothie	40
Sweet Potato Muffins	41
Edamame Frittata	42
Crustless Spinach Quiche	43

Chapter Four: SALADS & SOUPS 45

Crave-Worthy Egg Salad	46
Stuffed Avocado Salmon Salad	47
Avocado Chicken Salad	48
Pesto Chicken Salad	49
Butter Lettuce Salad with Shrimp	50
Kale and Quinoa Salad	51
Rustic Italian Salad	52
Taco Jar Salad	53
Rainbow Fields Salad	54
Wild Arugula, Spinach, and Steak Salad	55
Classic Tomato Soup and Grilled Cheese	57
Warm Lentil and Kale Soup	59
Easy Chicken Chili	60
Chicken and Wild Rice Soup	61
Broccoli Cream Soup	62
Delicata Squash Soup	63
Creamy Potato Soup	65
Simple Veggie Soup	66
Secret Ingredient Beef Chili	67
Tofu Miso Soup	68

Chapter Five: MAIN DISHES 71

One-Pan Chicken
and Chickpea Bake   72

Lemony Garlic Shrimp   73

Lentil and Quinoa "Meat"balls   74

One-Pot Beef and Broccoli   75

Rainbow Chard–Stuffed
Chicken Breasts   76

Slow-Cooked Pulled Pork   77

Half Noodle Lasagna   78

Baked Chicken Legs   79

Cumin Chicken and Black Beans   80

Almond-Crusted Cod   81

Roasted Veggie Wrap   82

Create Your Own Flatbread   83

Two-Pan Turkey Dinner   84

Cashew Chicken (or Tempeh)
Lettuce Wraps   85

Mahi-Mahi Fish Tacos   86

Lamb Kabobs   88

Spinach Parmesan
Spaghetti Squash   89

Pan-Seared Rainbow Trout   90

Easy Black Bean Burger   91

Mediterranean Roasted Salmon   92

Turkey Arugula Pasta   93

Tofu Stir-Fry   94

Sausage with Apple Sauerkraut
and Potatoes   95

Beef Stew   96

Savory Meatballs with Egg Noodles   97

Chapter Six: SIDES & SNACKS 99

Sides 100

Roasted Potatoes, Carrots,
and Asparagus   101

Roasted Broccoli with Shallots   102

Sweet Potato Fries   103

Shredded Brussels Sprouts,
Apples, and Pecans   104

Parmesan Green Beans and
Mushrooms   105

Simple Coleslaw   106

Three-Grain Ancient Blend   107

Cauliflower Mash   108

Fresh Veggie Couscous   109

Snacks 110

Turmeric Hummus   111

Peanut Butter Energy Bites   112

Berry Parfait   113

Roasted Chickpeas   114

Citrus Snack Plate   115

Mozzarella Bites   116

Traditional Caprese Salad   117

Home-Baked Kale Chips   119

Artichoke, Spinach,
and White Bean Dip   120

Classic Deviled Eggs   121

Chapter Seven: DRINKS & DESSERTS 123

Drinks 124

Knockout Nausea Water	125
Berry- and Basil-Infused Water	126
Electrolyte Balance	127
Caffeine-Free Vanilla Latte	128
Lactation Tea Blend	129
Sugar-Free Freshly Squeezed Lemonade	130
Pineapple Mojito Mocktail	131

Desserts 132

Strawberries and Cream	133
Dark Chocolate–Covered Raisins	134
Cinnamon Sugar Apples	135
Seedy Chocolate Bark	136
Avocado Chocolate Pudding	138
Mini Blueberry Pies	139
Lactation Cookies	140
Coconut Macaroons	141

Chapter Eight: EXTRAS 143

Nausea-Diffusing Blend	144
Relaxing Face Mask	145
Back Pain Relief Serum	146
Stretch Mark Cream	147
Zucchini Bread	148
Simple Go-To Salad Dressing	150

Resources	153
References	154
Index	156
Symptoms Index	165

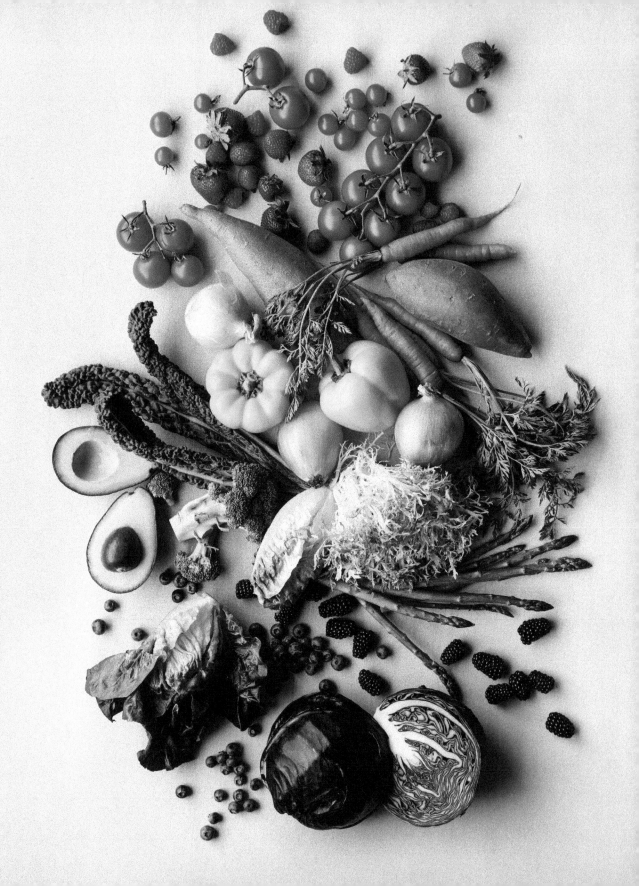

Introduction

WELCOME TO THE FEEL-GOOD PREGNANCY COOKBOOK! I'm so happy that I will be a part of your journey in a small way. My mission is to provide you with a holistic view of good health during pregnancy and beyond that is based on realistic, science-backed recommendations. This cookbook advances that mission by presenting easy and delicious go-to recipes that will provide good nutrition during this exciting time in your life.

In the three years I taught nutrition classes and provided one-on-one counseling to individuals participating in the Supplemental Nutrition Assistance Program, I was surprised to learn how little nutrition is discussed with pregnant women and new mothers. In fact, the extent of nutrition education at regular check-ups during pregnancy is typically a prenatal vitamin recommendation and sometimes a brief handout covering the foods pregnant women should avoid.

I decided to dedicate my entire practice to prenatal nutrition because I believe nutrition is the foundation of life and that everyone deserves a healthy, happy start. I love to teach people that nutrition doesn't have to be stressful and that finding balance and consistency is possible, especially during a time as special as pregnancy.

Even though information on nutrition is readily available, we still struggle to combat the world's leading preventable health conditions: obesity, heart disease, and diabetes. Consumers are more confused than ever about what to eat due to supplement industry messaging, the promotion of fad diets, and societal pressure to look a certain way. Recommendations are all over the place. Add pregnancy to the mix, and food choices get even foggier. Unfortunately, prenatal nutrition recommendations tend to be fear based, making pregnant women worry that anything they eat may affect their growing baby. One example is the warning against eating seafood due to its high mercury content, when in fact fish like salmon (check out the recipes on pages 47 and 92) are low in mercury and provide vital nutrients that are important for a baby's brain development. At a time when quality nutrition is more important than ever, women are eliminating a lot of nutritious foods from their diets. I'm here to tell you it does not have to be this way.

With this book, I hope to empower you with the tools and know-how you need to make confident decisions about the most nutritious foods to eat during your pregnancy. These recipes not only fuel a healthy pregnancy, but they are also easy to make and delicious to eat. Eating healthfully can be fun as well. Let's get started!

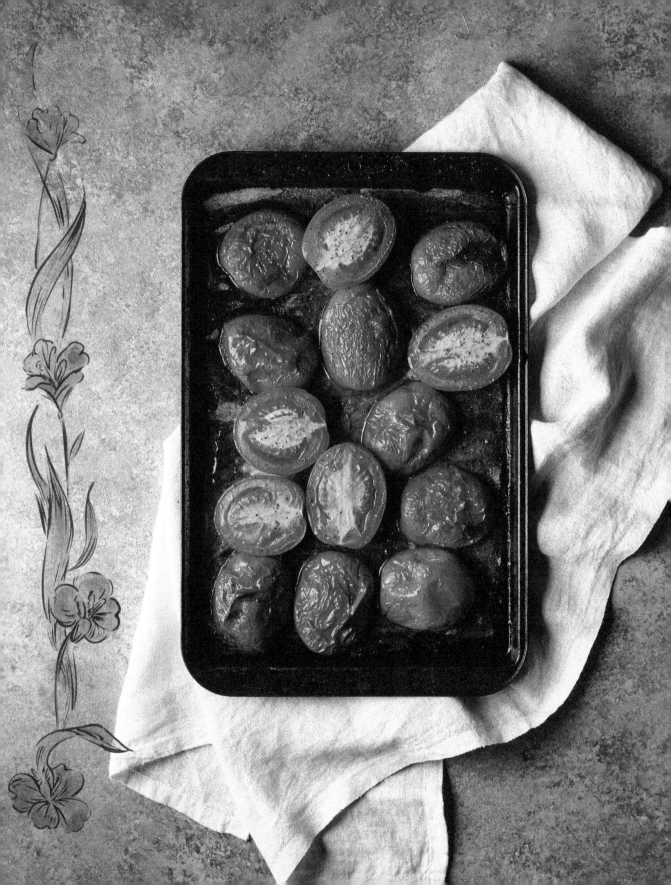

CHAPTER ONE

Feel Good,

PREGNANT

Pregnancy is an exciting but sometimes overwhelming experience. Although you may feel like everyone else is trying to direct your life and daily choices, rest assured that you are the one at the steering wheel, and you should be driving down the road of joy, comfort, and gratitude. You now have the amazing job of creating life.

Sharing your body is not an easy task, and that reality should not be underestimated. But feeling good and making time to be the best you is important! Happiness, like pregnancy, comes in all forms, shapes, and sizes. Do your pregnancy your way.

You're Pregnant!

To start, congratulations! You are growing a tiny human! Pregnancy is an unforgettable journey that is sure to make you stronger and wiser and ready to take on life's greatest adventures. Whether you found out today that you are pregnant or you are due tomorrow, you'll find insights in this book that will help you build confidence in your ability to nourish yourself and your baby. More than a cookbook, this book proposes an inventive, holistic approach to a healthy pregnancy. So, whether this is your first or fifth pregnancy, you will learn something new in these pages. I encourage you to use this book throughout your pregnancy and well beyond the day your baby is born.

We know that health is multifaceted, meaning many factors contribute to our well-being. Food, sleep, human connection, and physical activity all play a role in health. These factors remain relevant and could even be considered more important during pregnancy than at any other time of your life. Remember, good health for you ultimately means good health for your baby. What are a few traits that would describe the best version of you? Energized, strong, and happy? Know that it's never too late to take control of your health and become the best version of you. Achieving optimal health is a continuous, ever-evolving process.

Pregnancy doesn't come without its obstacles. There will be ups and downs, and sometimes you may feel that you are on a roller coaster. I'm here to tell you that the ups and downs are normal, thanks in large part to fluctuating pregnancy hormones. According to the March of Dimes, an estimated 70 percent of women experience morning sickness. Although queasiness often goes away in the second trimester, it can persist.

In addition to nausea, you may also experience heartburn, cramps, fatigue, and constipation. Some of these symptoms are hard to avoid, but it's important to focus on what you can do to abate them. Luckily, food—specifically some recipes in this book—will help you manage common pregnancy annoyances and discomforts.

Pregnancy brings some good, some bad, and many beautiful things to your life; make it a goal to enjoy every minute of it. If this isn't your first rodeo, recognize that every pregnancy can be very different. If this is your first rodeo, come to peace with the fact that you won't be able to control everything. Do your best with the resources and information you have available.

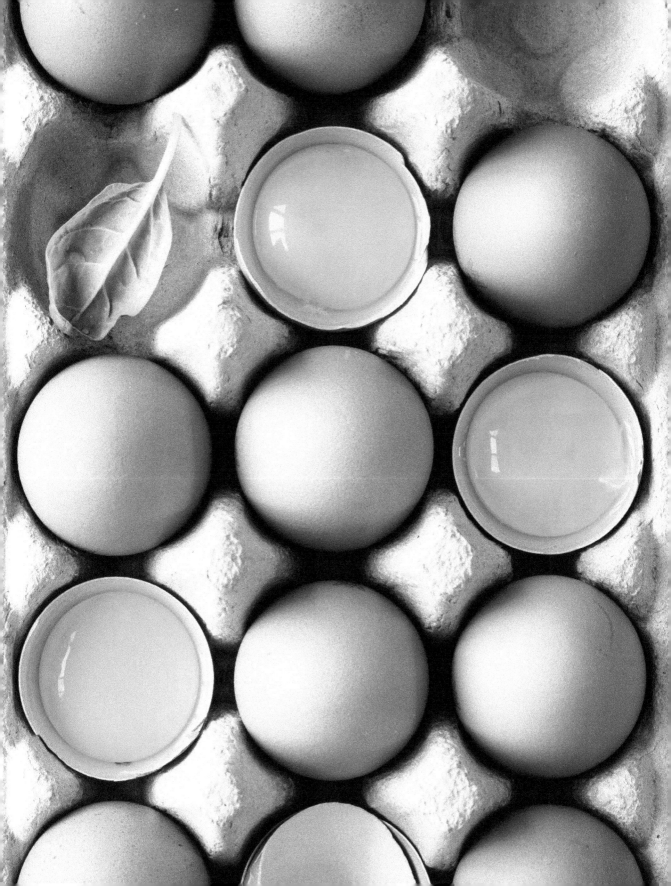

SELF-CARE

Self-care means doing things that make you feel happy, whole, and rejuvenated. During pregnancy, self-care is for you and your baby. Self-care decreases stress and anxiety, refreshes your mind and body, and helps you focus on just you for a moment.

So, how do you know if you need more self-care or need to start making self-care a part of your regular routine? For starters, if you are feeling so overwhelmed and busy that you can hardly come up for air, stop and take some time for yourself as soon as possible. Or if you often feel stressed, restless, or exhausted, you probably need to start carving out time each week to do something that is relaxing to you.

Self-care is important for everyone. If you feel like your life is just too hectic, I encourage you to look at your schedule and see if you can block out 10 minutes to stretch or close your eyes and take a few deep breaths. A little bit of self-care can go a long way. If you are someone who uses a planner to organize your days, write down "self-care" or what you will actually do for self-care. For example: "10:00 a.m., watch a funny cat video and laugh out loud." Another way to ensure you are getting in your self-care is to pick a day of the week to do something for yourself, such as "self-care Sunday."

Here are 10 ideas for self-care:

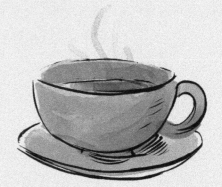

- Take a power nap
- Go for a walk and enjoy the fresh air
- Read your favorite book
- Get a facial or massage
- Take a workout class
- Write in a journal
- Make a green smoothie
- Go to brunch with friends
- See a therapist
- Snuggle with your pet

The beauty of self-care is that there are no rules or limitations surrounding it. It is going to look and feel different for everyone. Do what makes you feel good. Self-care is really about creating balance in your life. In order to take care of others, you have to first take care of yourself. This is even more true when you are expecting a baby.

Taking Care of You

It's no secret that the minute you become pregnant or give birth, the focus can shift from how you are doing to how the baby is doing. This is understandable and to be expected, but it's more than okay to take time for you! Keep in mind that taking care of you also means taking care of your baby. Listening to what feels like a million varying opinions about how you should be handling your pregnancy or birth can certainly be frustrating. Whether the advice is coming from friends, family, strangers, or your health-care team, it's crucial that you advocate for yourself and for the care you want and deserve.

What I'm saying is, this is your body, your pregnancy, and your baby! You are now not only in charge of your own health, but also a key player in the health of your baby. Write down any questions you might have and take them with you to your clinic. If you feel like something may be wrong, go in for an additional visit or schedule an appointment with a specialist. It's great if you have a partner with whom to share this journey, but remember, you are the only one who knows how you feel. Let your partner—and family members and friends—know what you desire. For example, let them know whether you prefer to be accompanied at doctor appointments or to go to them alone.

Let's talk about priorities. During this time you will be faced with a lot of tasks—for example, choosing a health-care provider, lining up a location to give birth, deciding who will be present at your baby's birth, and gathering must-have items prior to delivery. I encourage you to remember what is most important to you and to let go of some of the less important items on your to-do list. Taking care of yourself, including enjoying this book's nutrient-dense recipes, should be your priority. Remember that what you make a priority for yourself has a direct impact on your baby.

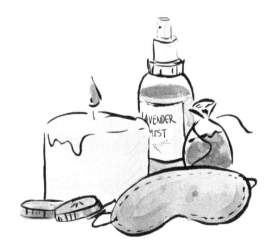

This Pregnancy: What to Expect

During pregnancy, your body will go through many wonderful changes to grow and develop your baby. Although you may not notice anything right away, changes are taking place as early as the first week of your pregnancy. Some of these changes may be expected and some unexpected, but don't worry—everything is taking place just as it should. The body is truly amazing. It knows exactly when to begin each milestone of pregnancy.

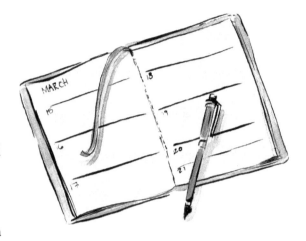

Your health-care provider has likely studied and worked with pregnant women for years, delivering thousands of healthy and happy babies. All questions are good questions, so don't be afraid to ask your provider. In fact, asking someone on your health-care team is much better than trusting information on the Internet, which is generally not a reliable source of information for most topics related to pregnancy. Instead, turn to licensed health professionals such as physical therapists, registered nurses, registered dietitians, or certified nurse-midwives—especially those who specialize in prenatal care.

What you eat plays a huge role in your pregnancy and should not be taken lightly. One of the biggest, mostly unavoidable changes that happens during pregnancy is weight gain. After all, you are growing a tiny human inside of you. But nutrition is a key component of your weight, just as it is for the average person who is not pregnant.

Although weight gain during pregnancy is completely expected and normal, health institutions have established certain prenatal weight guidelines. The key word here is "guidelines." Keep in mind that pregnant women will gain weight in different ways and possibly in different areas. How much weight you gain and where you gain it does not define your pregnancy as "healthy or unhealthy." Instead of focusing on that number on the scale, think about the foods you are eating each day. Eat healthy foods and the weight gain that is right for you should come naturally.

The following are brief descriptions of your baby's development throughout each trimester and what you may experience as a result.

FIRST TRIMESTER

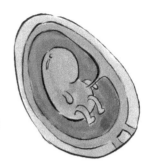

According to the Mayo Clinic, trimester one begins as
soon as you become pregnant and lasts until week 12.
Because so much is happening in your pregnancy each
week—the sex of your baby is actually determined as
soon as you conceive—providers often like to talk about
stages of pregnancy according to the week instead
of the month. Although your body experiences many
changes during weeks one through four, you may not notice signs of pregnancy
until weeks five through eight. These signs can include breast tenderness,
fatigue, and mood swings, all of which may last throughout the first trimester.

The hormones in your body are increasing and decreasing constantly, adjusting
to the work of building a baby. While you are going about your day-to-day life, complex processes are going on in your body. By week six, the baby's spinal cord has
closed over, the brain is growing, the heart is pumping, the digestive and respiratory
tracts are forming, and little bulbs that will turn into the baby's limbs have formed.

As this amazing development is occurring, you may begin to experience "morning sickness." Morning sickness is a misnomer because bouts of nausea can occur
at any point in the day. The exact cause is unknown, but morning sickness is likely
due to the rapid hormone changes that come with pregnancy. Nausea can range
from mild to severe, resulting in slight discomfort to frequent vomiting. Although
there is no "cure" for nausea, there are many things you can try to help reduce it.
One technique is to find an aroma you like—such as the Nausea-Diffusing Blend
of essential oils on page 144—and breathe it in when nausea hits. Sip water
throughout the day or eat small snacks to avoid having an empty stomach. Try
ginger tea or the Knockout Nausea Water on page 125. If you are vomiting, drink
a glass of the Electrolyte Balance drink on page 127. If you can figure out what
triggers your nausea, you can work to address it before it strikes.

Other changes to expect during the first trimester are breast growth to
prepare for milk production, minor spotting due to the placenta growing and
attaching to the uterus, more frequent urination, fatigue, and dizziness or headaches. Proper hydration, consumption of nutrient-dense foods, and appropriate
rest are all key in this phase of pregnancy.

By the end of the first trimester, your baby will start to look like a tiny person,
have functioning organ systems, and be around three inches long.

SECOND TRIMESTER

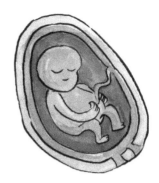

Week 13 marks the start of the second trimester. Between weeks 13 and 16, nausea and vomiting may subside, and you may begin to feel more like yourself again. You may even notice pregnancy glow—a real thing!—due to the large increase in blood flow created by the beating of two hearts inside of you.

At this point, the baby is able to move his or her arms and legs, but you may not feel them just yet. By week 16, the baby's reproductive system, hair, eyes, and ears have all formed more definitively.

Because your blood volume and blood flow increase to accommodate your baby, your iron needs increase. Most clinics routinely test for iron, and you may already be taking a supplement, but be sure to include iron in your diet as well. To boost your iron consumption, try Slow-Cooked Pulled Pork (page 77), Lamb Kabobs (page 88), and Beef Stew (page 96). You can get iron from both plant and animal sources, but keep in mind that your body is better able to absorb iron from animal sources.

Heartburn and constipation are two other symptoms you may start to experience as you get closer to the halfway point of pregnancy. Because your uterus is quickly expanding to keep up with the growth of your baby, your other organs are getting a bit squished, resulting in heartburn (indigestion), constipation, or both. Avoid spicy and greasy foods. Because chocolate may also increase heartburn, skip the Dark Chocolate–Covered Raisins (page 134), Avocado Chocolate Pudding (page 138), and Seedy Chocolate Bark (page 136) after the first trimester. Try going for a long walk after eating to kick-start digestion. If you are experiencing constipation, fiber and fluids are extra important. Try the Warm Lentil and Kale Soup (page 59), the Rainbow Fields Salad (page 54), the Shredded Brussels Sprouts, Apples, and Pecans side (page 104), or the Simple Veggie Soup (page 66). Keep in mind that some iron, calcium, and magnesium supplements can make constipation worse.

After passing the halfway point of your pregnancy, you will likely notice more rapid weight gain, possibly around one pound per week. Remember, this weight is due to the size of your baby, your breasts, the placenta, amniotic fluid, and increased blood volume. By the end of the second trimester, the baby's skin has thickened and the baby's fingerprints, lungs, liver, and immune system are almost completely formed. The baby's brain continues to develop rapidly, and the baby may be able to hear your voice.

THIRD TRIMESTER

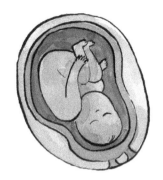

The final stretch! Week 28 marks the beginning of the third trimester. If you didn't notice an increase in your weight last trimester, you are likely to do so during the final months. The baby is putting on more layers of fat and gaining ounces each week. The rest of the reproductive organs develop, the lungs continue to mature, and a sleep and wake cycle is starting. Your baby's brain is now involved in complex bodily functions.

Common discomforts during this phase include leg cramps, back pain, and swelling. If you are experiencing cramps, swelling, or both, try drinking more water, invest in a good pair of shoes, and elevate your feet. Leg cramps may be a sign that you are not eating enough magnesium, potassium, sodium, or B vitamins. Try the Crustless Spinach Quiche (page 43) or the Avocado Chicken Salad (page 48) to increase these nutrients in your diet. If you are having back pain, try the Back Pain Relief Serum on page 146. You may also try a heated blanket and stretching to diminish the pain.

By week 33, the baby is mostly developed. You may gradually feel fewer movements from the baby because your uterus is very crowded at this point. At week 37, the baby is considered full term. All of your baby's systems are working better and better each day. Until your baby is born, you continue to provide your baby with antibodies and protein substances that help fight disease.

During this stage of pregnancy, take time to prepare your birth plan and decide how you will feed your baby. Classes about delivery, breastfeeding, and infant care are extremely helpful even if you are not a first-time mom. How you plan to feed your baby is ultimately your choice, but know that researchers have determined that the most optimal nutrition for infants is breast milk. Nursing is superior to formula in many ways. Breastfeeding benefits the mom, the baby, the family/partner, and the environment. Although it is scientifically impossible to replicate breast milk, advances in science and technology continually lead to better formulas.

As you get closer to your due date, you may notice some breast discharge, which is known as colostrum. Some women collect this milk so they can give it to their baby. It is packed with immune-boosting benefits.

You're ready! Breathe, relax, and trust yourself and your birth team. You can do this!

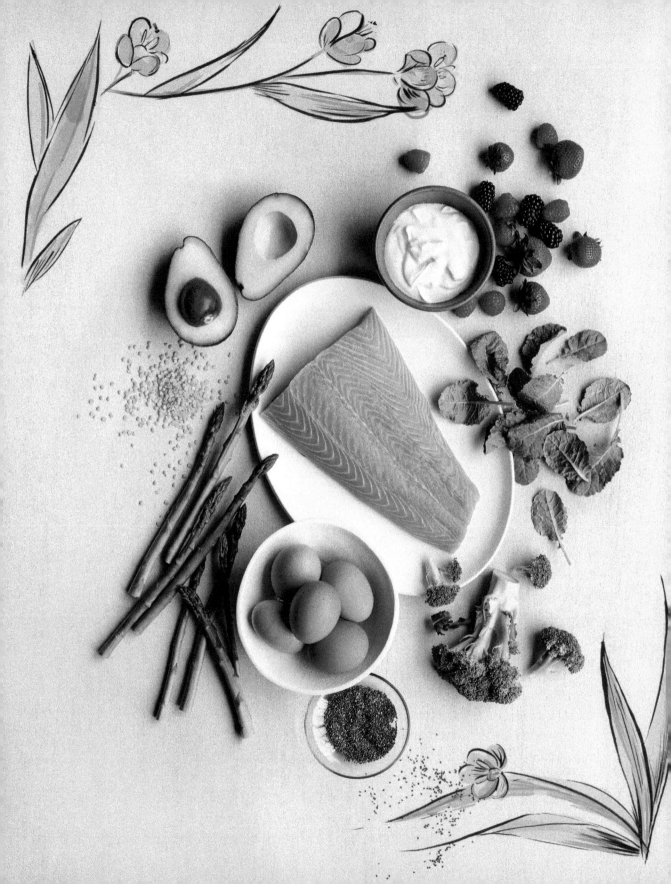

CHAPTER TWO

Figuring Out
WHAT TO EAT

Wading through often-conflicting nutrition advice can be challenging enough when you're not pregnant. Toss in the common pregnancy "food rules" and you end up with a little bit of chaos. This reality makes choosing healthy foods challenging each and every day. Know that there is no one-size-fits-all diet during pregnancy. Each pregnancy is unique and sometimes unpredictable, making it hard to always be on your nutrition A game. Keep in mind that planning is a big part of what makes healthy eaters successful. Maximize your nutrition each day you are feeling good, and don't be too hard on yourself if you don't get it just right all the time. The goal of this book is to help you determine the most nutritional diet for you and provide you with the tools and recipes you need to implement that diet.

What Do I (and Baby) Need?

The best answer is real food—food in its most whole form, grown in the earth, and minimally processed. This type of food seldom has a food label and is considered nutrient-dense rather than energy-dense. What is the difference? Energy-dense foods (such as potato chips) provide a lot of calories and few nutrients, whereas nutrient-dense foods (such as bell peppers) provide high amounts of nutrients with fewer calories.

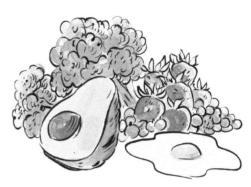

If you focus on eating a wide variety of real foods that have not been processed, you will get the nutrients you need for optimal health. Keep in mind that we eat food, not nutrients. That's why it's best to make thoughtful choices about the foods you are including in your diet instead of aiming for specific nutrient amounts. Foods contain a multitude of nutrients that work together to maintain your body's health.

That said, your health care team may recommend that you take dietary supplements during your pregnancy. Supplements are meant to serve as an insurance policy; they can help if you have severe food allergies and have to eliminate certain food groups, or if you have nausea and vomiting. But when taken on their own, some nutrients have different effects on our health compared to when they are consumed naturally in foods. For this reason, I highly encourage you to get the bulk of your nutrition through real food and not supplements.

NO NEED TO EAT FOR TWO

In case you haven't heard, "eating for two" is a myth—however, nourishment for two is very real. You are your baby's direct source of nutrition. A study published in 2010 by University of California, Davis, researchers Janet Uriu-Adams and Carl Keen even suggests that what you eat during pregnancy affects your grandchildren. No worries, though; the information and recipes in this book are sure to make your pregnancy journey a positive and healthy one for generations to come.

AVOID PROCESSED FOODS

Limit processed foods as much as possible. For example:

- chips
- cereals
- snack crackers like goldfish
- foods labeled "instant"
- bagels
- pretzels
- pizza
- boxed pasta or other foods with refined carbohydrates

Other foods to limit are those high in added sugar such as:

- sweets and pastries
- soda
- fruit juice
- sports drinks
- energy drinks
- bottled teas
- blended coffee beverages
- dipping sauces like barbeque sauce, ketchup, teriyaki, and honey mustard
- fruit yogurts
- granola
- protein bars
- bottled smoothies
- canned fruit

WHAT SPECIFIC NUTRIENTS FUEL A HEALTHY PREGNANCY?

All of the food groups are necessary to properly fuel you and your baby. Fat, protein, and carbohydrates (carbs) all play a pivotal role in maintaining your health during pregnancy and promoting the growth of your baby. However, fat is often mistakenly associated with weight gain, even though the fat you eat doesn't correlate to gaining more or less weight during pregnancy. There are many factors that contribute to how much weight women gain when they are pregnant, which is why adopting a low-fat diet won't result in fewer extra pounds. Adequate fat consumption during pregnancy is so important because your need for the fat-soluble vitamins A, D, E, and K increases. These vitamins support proper development of your baby's brain, eyes, bones, heart, and immune function. If you don't eat enough fat, you will likely be deficient in these essential nutrients, so don't fear chicken skins or fatty meats like pulled pork, full-fat dairy, or plant fats such as nuts, seeds, olives, and coconut.

Adequate protein consumption is also critical during pregnancy, as every new cell that is produced in your developing baby needs this nutrient. Protein will help keep you full, provide you with energy, potentially prevent headaches, and help balance your blood sugar. Eat a variety of protein-rich foods, including those from animals and plants.

Lastly, you should incorporate healthy carbs, such as sweet potatoes, into your diet. Other options include fruit, corn, peas, squash, milk or yogurt, legumes, and ancient grains. Since carbs are the only food group that can significantly raise your blood sugar, it's very important to pay attention to both the quality and the amount of carbs you eat. A 2016 study published in *Nutrients* and a 2014 study published in the *Journal of Nutrition & Intermediary Metabolism* collectively suggest that higher weight gain, larger babies, increased risk of gestational diabetes and preeclampsia, and other negative pregnancy-related outcomes occur with higher carb intake. That being said, everyone tolerates a different amount of carbs in their diet, and it is crucial to pair your carbs with a source of fat and/or protein (for example, eating an apple with almonds as opposed to an apple by itself). It is wise to get your blood sugar checked by your doctor regularly, even before your test for gestational diabetes, if possible.

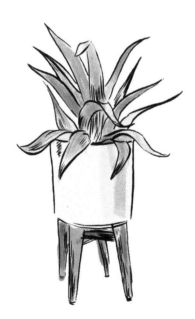

TOP 10 FOODS

Variety is important when it comes to your prenatal diet, and the intent of this list isn't to limit your food options. There are plenty of foods outside of this list that provide excellent nutrition for you and your baby. Also, keep in mind that there are no "superfoods" that will ensure you have a perfect pregnancy. The foods listed below are in no particular order and all contain nutrients considered to be an important part of your and your baby's health during pregnancy.

1. **Salmon:** Salmon, preferably wild-caught, provides approximately 1,400 mg of DHA, an omega-3 fatty acid that is crucial for the development of your baby's brain. It is estimated that you need around 300 mg of DHA per day, although research published in the *Archives of Disease in Childhood: Fetal and Neonatal Edition* in 2008 suggests more than 300 mg is beneficial. Getting direct sources of DHA—not ALA—is essential. The other good news is that salmon is also one of the few dietary sources of vitamin D. It contains selenium, iodine, and zinc as well, which contribute to the overall growth of your baby and help develop your baby's reproductive organs.

2. **Eggs:** Eggs provide a nutrient known as choline, which is similar to folate in function. Both of these important nutrients help develop your baby's brain and spinal cord in the first several weeks of pregnancy. Choline is also involved in building your baby's DNA. Most of the choline, and a good amount of the other nutrients eggs provide, are in the yolk, so be sure to eat the whole thing. If you are a vegetarian, eggs should be incorporated into your diet daily.

3. **Berries:** Berries are a great source of fiber and antioxidants. Blackberries provide 8 g of fiber per cup. Strawberries contain some folate, too. Berries are a good fruit to eat if you have gestational diabetes.

4. **Chia seeds:** Chia seeds contain ideal quantities of fiber and a variety of minerals such as iron, calcium, and magnesium. They are included in the Berry Parfait on page 113 but can also be an excellent addition to smoothies, oatmeal, and salads.

5. **Kale:** In general, leafy greens are important to include in your prenatal diet because of their folate content, but they also contain vitamins C and K, antioxidants, B vitamins, magnesium, potassium, and more. Again, adequate folate is needed to develop your baby's brain and spinal cord. A lot of women find the easiest way to get their greens is in a smoothie, which may help during times of severe nausea. Try the Protein-Packed Strawberry Smoothie on page 37. Kale is also worth trying cooked in dishes such as the Warm Lentil and Kale Soup (page 59).

6. **Greek yogurt:** Yogurt provides calcium, iodine, B vitamins, probiotics, protein, and vitamins A, D, E, and K. Greek yogurt provides additional protein and may be better tolerated by those who are sensitive to dairy. The probiotics in yogurt also promote the growth of healthy bacteria in your gut.

7. **Asparagus:** Asparagus is another non-starchy vegetable that provides natural folate and fiber. It also contains vitamins K, E, and C and copper. Try the Roasted Potatoes, Carrots, and Asparagus recipe on page 101 for an easy and delicious side dish that includes asparagus.

8. **Lentils:** Lentils provide protein, iron, folate, phosphorus, zinc, manganese, and copper, which makes them a great source of nutrition for vegetarians. Lentils and other legumes are high in carbohydrates, though, so be careful if you have gestational diabetes.

9. **Avocado:** Avocados are a great addition to your pregnancy diet. They are a good source of magnesium, fiber, B vitamins, vitamins K and E, and folate. Avocados contain healthy monounsaturated fats, so they help with the absorption of fat-soluble vitamins in leafy greens.

10. **Broccoli:** Broccoli is high in magnesium, calcium, and vitamins C, K, and A and contains small amounts of choline and folate. It is a versatile ingredient and can be used in the kitchen in many ways. Include more broccoli in your diet by trying the Roasted Broccoli with Shallots on page 102, the Cheesy Mini Quiches on page 30, and the Broccoli Cream Soup on page 62.

What Changes through the Months?

Focusing on a real-food diet throughout your pregnancy will keep you energized and help your baby thrive for a full nine months. You may notice frequent changes in your appetite, which is completely normal. Take the time to learn about your body and listen to the cues it gives you. You'll be surprised how intuitive your body is at letting you know what you and your baby need.

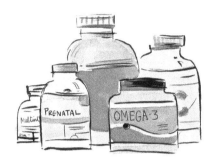

THE FIRST HALF OF PREGNANCY

Although nutrient needs increase in pregnancy, only a slight increase in overall calories is necessary. This is why it's important to focus on nutrient-dense foods versus a target calorie goal. Your calorie needs remain the same during the first few months of pregnancy, and you may even struggle to get those calories in due to morning sickness. Eat what you can keep down. It's okay if you end up eating more carbs in the first trimester, as this is what your body usually tolerates. Once you feel better, make it count.

Key nutrients during the first half of pregnancy include folate, choline, magnesium, DHA, and vitamins A, B_6, B_{12}, and D. Calcium needs do not increase, and absorption actually improves during pregnancy. Include one to two servings of greens daily, fatty fish twice per week, plus other quality proteins such as eggs, chicken, and beef, aged cheese and yogurt, and nuts and seeds.

THE SECOND HALF OF PREGNANCY

Calorie and protein needs increase in the second half of pregnancy. As you head into the second trimester, you may benefit from adding in an extra snack each day. Throughout the second half of pregnancy, 250 to 500 additional calories are needed per day. Try adding a Mango Carrot Smoothie (page 38) or the Peanut Butter Energy Bites (page 112) to your usual meals.

Key nutrients during the second half of pregnancy include iron, zinc, glycine (an amino acid in protein), vitamins E and K, and probiotics. Eat a rainbow of vegetables and fruits, try fermented vegetables, and add in slow-cooked meats such as beef stew (check out the recipe on page 96). Add extra calories to your meals by choosing full-fat dairy, eating the skin on meats, adding extra avocado, or using real butter or animal fat when cooking. Keep in mind that the nutrients that were noted as important during the first half of pregnancy remain important throughout your entire pregnancy.

SPECIAL CONCERNS

As mentioned previously, pregnancy has an interesting way of throwing various curveballs. Some curveballs include gestational diabetes or a twin pregnancy, which may warrant additional nutritional support and guidance. I've included some info below. Do not worry though—there are many experts eagerly waiting to help you on this journey and answer all the questions you have.

GESTATIONAL DIABETES MELLITUS (GDM)

GDM testing is typically completed between weeks 24 and 28 of pregnancy. If you have been diagnosed with GDM, meet with a registered dietitian to figure out the amount of carbs that is right for you. It's important to check your blood sugar regularly to ensure it never gets too high. Be sure to eat plenty of foods rich in protein, magnesium, and vitamin D, and consider supplementation if needed.

MULTIPLES

If you are pregnant with twins or more, your overall calorie and protein needs are even higher. Follow the tips listed in The Second Half of Pregnancy section to add extra calories to your meals and snacks. Consult with a prenatal nutrition specialist if you are unsure if you are eating the correct amount for you.

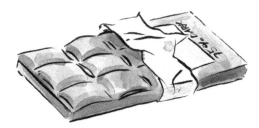

SPECIAL DIETS

Many women follow specific diets or lifestyles before they get pregnant, and it's only natural for moms-to-be to want to continue eating as they have in the past. Specific diets may include vegetarian, vegan, pescatarian, dairy-free, gluten-free, paleo, or keto. As soon as you know you're pregnant, have a conversation with your health-care team about your nutritional needs during pregnancy. Now more than ever it's important to make sure you are getting all the nutrients your growing baby needs to thrive. Work with your doctor or a licensed nutritionist to adjust your diet as needed.

VEGETARIAN

As a vegetarian, you will have to make some dietary adjustments to ensure you are getting enough iron, zinc, vitamin A (specifically the form known as "retinol" that's found in animal products), vitamin B_{12}, vitamin K, choline, glycine, and DHA. The amino acid glycine becomes conditionally essential in pregnancy—meaning you have to get it through your diet—and it is only found in meat. Vitamin B_{12} is also solely found in animal products. Due to the bioavailability of iron and zinc in plant foods (i.e., to what degree these nutrients are absorbed by the body), vegetarians often need more than what they are able to consume. To ensure adequate nutrition, pregnant vegetarians should eat eggs and dairy daily, and take a high-quality prenatal vitamin with a direct source of DHA. Talk with a registered dietitian about other nutrient needs to consider if you plan to continue eating a vegetarian diet during pregnancy. A 2019 study published in *Nutrients* concluded that plant-based diets are safe during pregnancy as long as macronutrient and micronutrient needs are met, which does take careful consideration and dietary management.

VEGAN

Many choose the vegan lifestyle out of a strong opposition to eating animals or animal products. Others become vegan for health reasons. If you decide to continue a vegan diet during your pregnancy, be sure to consult with a prenatal nutrition specialist or a functional medicine physician about what you can do to ensure your baby is getting the necessary nutrients to thrive. Taking supplements may be recommended, but also see page 12 for a discussion of the importance of food over supplements.

PESCATARIAN

Pescatarians likely consume plenty of DHA through the fish they eat, which is great for a baby's developing brain and eyes. However, pescatarians may not obtain enough glycine in their regular diet, and their potential risk for taking in too much mercury is higher than for those who don't eat as much fish. Focus on smaller fish such as sardines, herring, salmon, cod, shrimp, trout, and halibut to avoid excess mercury. If you are adventurous, try salmon roe. Also, be sure to include plenty of eggs and dairy in your diet.

DAIRY-FREE

Many follow a dairy-free diet because of allergies or lactose intolerance. Pregnant women who follow a dairy-free diet still need the nutrients dairy products provide, such as protein, calcium, iodine, vitamins K and D, B vitamins, and probiotics. Other sources of these nutrients include almonds, sardines, salmon, broccoli, leafy greens, chia and sesame seeds, and fermented vegetables like sauerkraut.

GLUTEN-FREE

You likely won't have any problems meeting your nutrient needs by eliminating gluten alone. Gluten-free grains such as amaranth, millet, teff, brown rice, and quinoa can be included in your diet.

PALEO

The "caveman" diet has the potential to be a healthy option during pregnancy since the emphasis is on eating whole foods and avoiding processed items. However, this diet typically eliminates dairy, grains, and legumes that, in combination, provide probiotics, iodine, calcium, vitamins K and D, B vitamins, fiber, iron, and valuable energy. A modified paleo diet that includes full-fat dairy and ancient grains is a more well-rounded approach.

KETO

I do not recommend a diet that eliminates carbs completely. As discussed on page 13, all of the food groups contribute to the health of you and your baby. However, diets lower in carbs may be beneficial for some, especially those with GDM.

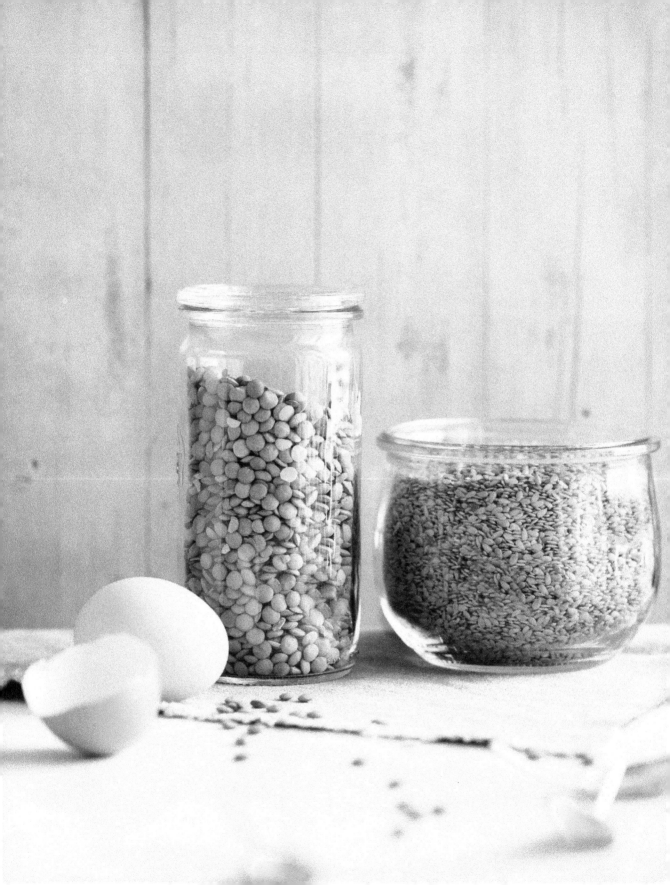

How to Use This Book

This book is designed so that you can try certain recipes as they fit into your lifestyle throughout your pregnancy and beyond. I encourage you to first flip through it to get a taste (no pun intended) of the types of recipes that are included. The format follows that of a traditional cookbook for ease of use. Each recipe includes information about how much the recipe makes, the nutritional breakdown of each serving, the time you'll spend preparing and cooking the recipe from start to finish, an ingredients list, detailed directions, and sometimes a bonus tip to help you alter or enhance the recipe.

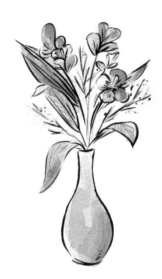

FINDING THE RIGHT RECIPES FOR YOU

Recipe labels will help you determine whether a recipe suits your dietary needs or may lessen one of your symptoms. They specify which recipes are good for conception, postpartum recovery, or lactation.

Labels include:

DIETARY NEEDS

- Dairy-Free: recipes free of any product made from a cow

- Gluten-Free: recipes free of wheat, rye, and barley

- Nut-Free: no nuts included

- Soy-Free: recipes free of soy and soy products

- Vegetarian: no meat, fish, or poultry included

- Vegan: no animal products included

SYMPTOMS AND LIFESTYLE

- Energy Enhancer: try these recipes to increase your energy

- Gestational Diabetes–Friendly: lower in carbs and unlikely to spike your blood sugar

- Good for Constipation: recipes high in fiber

- Good for Lactation: good for enhancing the quality of your breast milk or boosting your milk supply

- Good for Leg Cramps: recipes that help relieve cramps

- Good for Nausea: recipes that are higher in B_6 and magnesium or that contain ginger

- Good for Postpartum Recovery: will help replenish your body after you've given birth

- Good for Pre-Conception: helpful if you are currently trying to conceive

- Good for Swelling: may help reduce your chances of swelling or reduce swelling

- Kid-Friendly: recipes your kids will also love

- May Help with Headaches: recipes worth trying if you have frequent headaches

- Quick: recipes made in under 30 minutes

LOCATING RECIPES BY SYMPTOM

Good nutrition can help with many of the discomforts that come with pregnancy, including nausea, swelling, leg cramps, headaches, and more. Refer to the Symptoms Index (page 165) to find recipes that are organized according to the pregnancy symptoms they address. (The general Index [page 156] will help you navigate the book more broadly.) Eating during pregnancy should still be enjoyable, regardless of your symptoms. How does Blueberry Pecan Pancakes (page 28) for breakfast, Rainbow Fields Salad (page 54) for lunch, and Slow-Cooked Pulled Pork (page 77) for dinner sound? The recipes in this book will supply you with the nutrition you need to feel good!

WHAT YOU'LL NEED TO GET STARTED

Below are some of the items commonly used in the recipes in this book. Stock your pantry with these key ingredients:

FOOD

- Extra-virgin olive oil—good for dressings, pesto, and to top veggies

- Avocado oil—good for cooking at higher temperatures

- Grass-fed butter or ghee without added vegetable oil

- Coconut oil spray—good for greasing baking sheets and dishes, sauté pans, and skillets

- Seasonings such as salt, pepper, Italian seasoning, ginger, etc.

- Flour—coconut, almond, oat, or whole wheat

- Eggs—pasture-raised or organic, if feasible for you

KITCHEN EQUIPMENT

- Blender or food processor

- Medium-size pots and pans

- Cast-iron skillet—good for improving the iron content in foods

- Mixing bowls

- Glass food storage containers

- Round or square glass baking dishes

- Baking/cookie sheet

- Kitchen thermometer

Due to the risk of exposure to potentially harmful toxins contained in non-stick cookware, it is best to stick with glass, ceramic, stainless steel, or cast-iron cooking equipment and utensils. For more information regarding this topic, visit the Environmental Working Group website (www.ewg.org).

FOOD SAFETY TIPS

Food safety may not be something that is usually on your mind, but it deserves attention during pregnancy because contracting foodborne illnesses can be especially dangerous for pregnant women. When you are pregnant, your immune system is weakened, making it easier for you to get sick. Eating a well-rounded diet can strengthen your immune system, but practicing good food safety protocols will also help you avoid getting sick. Next are several tips for improving your safety around food.

1. **Wash your hands frequently.** Wash before and after handling food and eating, after taking out the trash, after touching any animal or animal product, and after using the bathroom.

2. **Avoid washing raw meat.**

3. **Use separate meat and produce cutting boards.**

4. **Use a meat thermometer to ensure your meats are cooked all the way through.** Heat all luncheon and deli meats. As a general rule, ensure all meats and fish reach 165°F.

5. **Wash all produce, even if it has a peel or has been labeled "pre-washed."**

6. **Throw away refrigerated leftovers within three to four days.**

7. **Avoid pre-made dishes or pre-cut produce at the store.** For example, buy a whole pineapple instead of diced pineapple in a plastic container.

8. **Avoid unpasteurized dairy products.**

9. **Avoid raw or undercooked shellfish.**

10. **Keep your kitchen tidy.** Clean your dishes and cooking equipment thoroughly, and ensure your refrigerator is organized to prevent cross-contamination. If you follow these recommendations, your risk of contracting an infection is low.

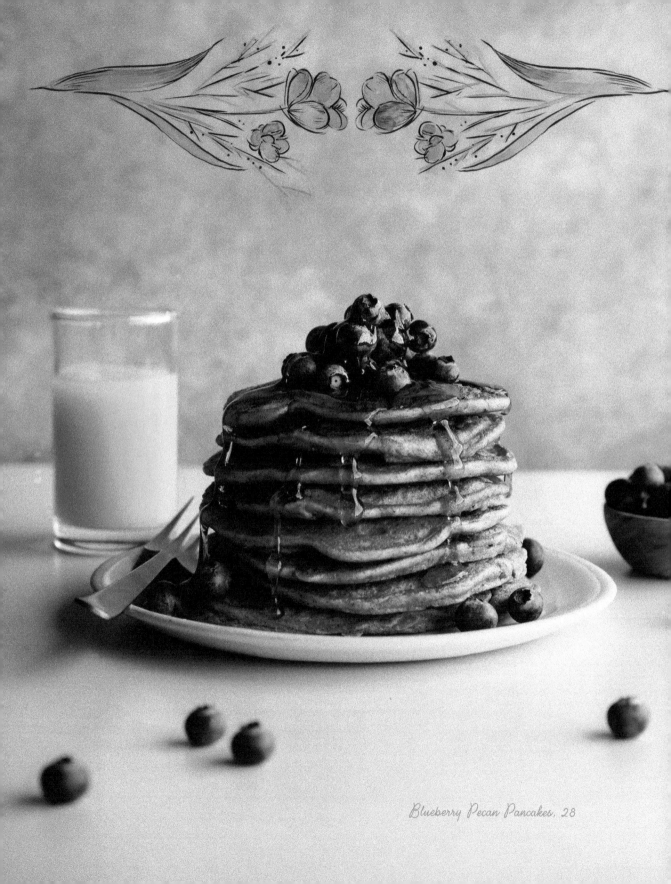

Blueberry Pecan Pancakes, 28

CHAPTER THREE

BREAKFAST

Breakfast—my favorite meal of the day—is a very important meal for a few reasons. First, it can actually help prevent morning sickness, which is not helped by an empty stomach. Second, it supplies nutrients to your baby after 12 hours of fasting in the evening. Third, breakfast gives you the energy you need to start your day, enhance your mood, and help balance your calories throughout the remainder of your day.

BLUEBERRY PECAN PANCAKES

....

Prep time: 5 minutes | Cook time: 25 minutes

Pancakes are one of my favorite breakfast foods, but they are often packed with sugar and refined carbs. This recipe is a bit healthier and even contains protein and antioxidants!

....

Yield: 10 to 12 (3-inch) pancakes

Serving size: 3 pancakes

GLUTEN-FREE, SOY-FREE, VEGETARIAN, KID-FRIENDLY

3 large eggs
1 teaspoon vanilla extract
½ cup milk
1 cup almond flour
1 tablespoon coconut sugar
   or other sugar
1 teaspoon cinnamon
½ teaspoon baking powder
½ teaspoon baking soda
2 scoops protein powder
¼ cup chopped pecans
1 tablespoon butter or
   coconut oil
1 pint fresh blueberries
Butter, for serving (optional)
Maple syrup or peanut butter
   (optional)

Per serving: Calories: 387; Total fat: 22g; Saturated fat: 5g; Carbohydrate: 27g; Sugar: 16g; Fiber: 6g; Protein: 22g; Sodium: 275mg; Cholesterol: 165mg

1. In a large bowl, combine the eggs, vanilla, and milk.

2. In a separate medium bowl, combine the flour, sugar, cinnamon, baking powder, baking soda, and protein powder.

3. Add the dry ingredients to the wet ingredients, stirring until just combined.

4. Mix in the pecans.

5. Heat the butter in a large sauté pan over medium heat.

6. Use a ladle to pour the batter into the hot pan, making each pancake approximately 3 inches in diameter. Place 5 to 7 blueberries in a random fashion on the surface of each pancake.

7. Once the surface of the pancakes begins to bubble (2 to 3 minutes), flip the pancakes and cook for another 1 to 2 minutes longer.

8. Top the pancakes with butter and a drizzle of maple syrup or peanut butter, if using.

Tip: Use almond milk to make the pancakes dairy-free and leave out the pecans to make them nut-free. Make a double batch of this recipe and freeze the second batch to use for breakfast on a busy weekday. The batter will last about 2 days in the refrigerator and the frozen pancakes for about 3 months. Place the frozen pancakes in the refrigerator before you go to bed to enjoy the next morning.

Carrot Cake for Breakfast

Prep time: 8 minutes | Cook time: 3 minutes

I love the idea of having a serving of veggies for breakfast. Adding carrots to oatmeal is the perfect way to enjoy a delicious breakfast while working toward your daily veggie goals.

Yield: 1 serving

Serving size: 1 cup

DAIRY-FREE, GOOD FOR LACTATION, KID-FRIENDLY

½ cup uncooked steel-cut oats

1 tablespoon pumpkin purée

2 teaspoons maple syrup

1 teaspoon vanilla extract

1 teaspoon cinnamon

1 small carrot, grated

½ cup unsweetened almond milk

1 tablespoon chopped walnuts

Pinch unsweetened coconut flakes (optional)

1 tablespoon raisins (optional)

Per serving: Calories: 472; Total fat: 12g; Saturated fat: 1g; Carbohydrate: 78g; Sugar: 13g; Fiber: 13g; Protein: 14g; Sodium: 132mg; Cholesterol: 0mg

1. Place the oats in a microwavable cereal bowl.

2. In a separate small bowl, combine the pumpkin purée, maple syrup, vanilla, cinnamon, and carrot.

3. Add the milk to the bowl with the oats and microwave it for about 3 minutes.

4. Stir the pumpkin mixture into the warmed oats.

5. Top with the walnuts and add coconut flakes or raisins, if using.

Tip: If you are experiencing frequent hunger, especially in the third trimester, add more protein and calories by using whole milk. Just note, it won't be dairy-free.

Cheesy Mini Quiches

Prep time: 15 minutes | Cook time: 20 minutes

These mini quiches are perfect for when you are having family or girlfriends over for a holiday or long weekend. They are easy to whip up but make you look like a fancy chef.

Yield: 12 quiches

Serving size:

1 to 2 quiches

NUT-FREE, SOY-FREE, VEGETARIAN, GOOD FOR POSTPARTUM RECOVERY, GOOD FOR PRE-CONCEPTION, KID-FRIENDLY

Coconut oil spray

1 pie crust dough sheet

6 large eggs, beaten

¼ cup milk

Salt

Freshly ground black pepper

½ cup shredded Cheddar cheese

1 cup broccoli, chopped

1. Preheat the oven to 400°F. Lightly spray a muffin tin with oil.

2. Roll out the pie crust and press the rim of a drinking glass into the dough to cut out 12 (2½-inch) muffin-size circles.

3. Place each dough cutout in the muffin tin.

4. In a large bowl, whisk together the eggs, milk, salt, and pepper.

5. Add the cheese.

6. Divide the egg mixture evenly between the muffin cups with the dough cutouts, filling each one about two-thirds full.

7. Divide the broccoli pieces between the muffin cups.

8. Bake in the oven for 20 minutes or until the edges of the crusts turn a nice golden brown.

Per serving: Calories: 219; Total fat: 15g; Saturated fat: 5g; Carbohydrate: 12g; Sugar: 2g; Fiber: 1g; Protein: 10g; Sodium: 293mg; Cholesterol: 174mg

Chorizo-Potato Hash

Prep time: 10 minutes | Cook time: 20 minutes

Who doesn't love a good breakfast hash? Chorizo is super flavorful, so this dish is sure to wake up your taste buds.

Yield: 3 servings

Serving size: 1 egg with 1 cup chorizo mixture

DAIRY-FREE, GLUTEN-FREE, NUT-FREE, SOY-FREE, QUICK

2 tablespoons avocado oil, divided
4 cups red potatoes, diced
½ small yellow onion, chopped
1 yellow bell pepper, seeded and chopped
7 to 9 ounces chorizo sausage
3 large eggs
Salt, for seasoning
Freshly ground black pepper, for seasoning

Per serving: Calories: 492; Total fat: 31g; Saturated fat: 9g; Carbohydrate: 39g; Sugar: 5g; Fiber: 4g; Protein: 21g; Sodium: 846mg; Cholesterol: 218mg

1. Heat 1 tablespoon of oil in a cast-iron skillet over medium heat. Add the potatoes and cook for 2 minutes before adding the onion. Cook for another 5 minutes.

2. Add the bell pepper and cook for an additional 5 minutes.

3. Add the chorizo and cook until the chorizo is browned and the potatoes are soft, 8 to 10 minutes.

4. Heat the remaining tablespoon of oil in a separate medium skillet over medium heat.

5. Fry the eggs and season them with salt and pepper.

6. Transfer the chorizo and potato mixture to three plates and top each serving with one of the eggs.

Tip: To make this recipe even faster, use a bag of frozen potatoes, peppers, and onions. Eliminate steps 1, 2, and 4 and add the whole bag to the skillet at the same time.

Egg in Tomato Bake

Prep time: 5 minutes | Cook time: 25 minutes

So simple yet so delicious, this dish reminds me of something you would eat in the Mediterranean.

Yield: 4 tomato egg bakes
Serving size: 1 to 2 tomato egg bakes

DAIRY-FREE, GLUTEN-FREE, VEGETARIAN, GESTATIONAL DIABETES–FRIENDLY, GOOD FOR PRE-CONCEPTION, GOOD FOR SWELLING

4 large beefsteak tomatoes
4 large eggs
1 tablespoon Italian seasoning
Salt, for seasoning
Freshly ground black pepper, for seasoning
2 tablespoons extra-virgin olive oil
1 medium avocado, pitted, peeled, and quartered (optional)

1. Preheat the oven to 425°F.

2. Cut the top off each tomato and scoop out the insides. Place the tomatoes, cut-side up, in a baking dish or pan.

3. Break each egg separately into a small bowl then pour it into a tomato until all the tomatoes are filled with an egg. Sprinkle the tomatoes with Italian seasoning, salt, pepper, and olive oil.

4. Bake for 25 minutes or until the eggs are fully cooked.

5. Top each tomato with a quarter of the avocado, if using.

Per serving: Calories: 333; Total fat: 26g; Saturated fat: 5g; Carbohydrate: 16g; Sugar: 11g; Fiber: 4g; Protein: 14g; Sodium: 143mg; Cholesterol: 332mg

Open-Face Egg Sandwich

Prep time: 10 minutes | Cook time: 10 minutes

Honestly, this is my go-to breakfast. You can whip it up on a busy morning.

Yield: 1 sandwich

Serving size: 1 sandwich

NUT-FREE, SOY-FREE, VEGETARIAN, ENERGY ENHANCER, QUICK

1 teaspoon extra-virgin olive oil

1 large egg

Salt, for seasoning

Freshly ground black pepper, for seasoning

1 cup raw spinach

1 whole-wheat bread slice, toasted

½ mini avocado or ¼ large avocado, peeled, pitted, and sliced

½ cup sautéed red bell pepper slices (optional)

Per serving: Calories: 251; Total fat: 17g; Saturated fat: 3g; Carbohydrate: 17g; Sugar: 2g; Fiber: 6g; Protein: 11g; Sodium: 376mg; Cholesterol: 164mg

1. Heat the oil in a small sauté pan over medium-low heat. Crack the egg into a small bowl, then add it to the pan.

2. Season the egg with salt and pepper and top it with the spinach.

3. Cook the egg for 3 to 5 minutes on both sides.

4. Once the egg is fully cooked, remove it from the pan and place it on the toasted bread. Top with the avocado slices and bell pepper slices, if using.

Tip: If you are extra hungry (as you might be in the second half of pregnancy or when breastfeeding), add two eggs instead of one. Enjoy with a side of strawberries or a juicy orange.

Egg, Bacon, and Veggie Breakfast Bake

Prep time: 15 minutes | Cook time: 40 to 45 minutes

This recipe is great if you want to have a veggie-filled breakfast that's easy to make ahead and heat up in the morning.

Yield: 12 servings

Serving size:
1 (2-inch) piece

GLUTEN-FREE, NUT-FREE, SOY-FREE, ENERGY ENHANCER, GESTATIONAL DIABETES–FRIENDLY, GOOD FOR POSTPARTUM RECOVERY, GOOD FOR SWELLING, KID-FRIENDLY

5 bacon slices
1 bell pepper, seeded and diced
3 cups shredded Brussels sprouts
1 tablespoon minced garlic
12 large eggs
½ cup milk

1. Preheat the oven to 400°F.

2. In a large skillet over medium heat, cook the bacon for approximately 8 minutes. When fully cooked, transfer the bacon to a paper towel–lined plate to drain.

3. In the same skillet, add the bell pepper, Brussels sprouts, and garlic, cooking until the garlic is browned and the veggies are tender, 10 to 15 minutes.

4. Crack all the eggs into a large bowl and add the milk.

5. Beat with a hand mixer or whisk (if you want a little arm workout).

6. When the bacon has cooled, chop it into small pieces.

7. In a 9-by-13-inch pan, evenly distribute the bacon and veggie mixture. Pour the egg mixture into the pan.

8. Bake for 20 minutes or until a kitchen thermometer shows the internal temperature has reached 160°F.

Per serving: Calories: 125; Total fat: 8g; Saturated fat: 3g; Carbohydrate: 4g; Sugar: 2g; Fiber: 1g; Protein: 10g; Sodium: 255mg; Cholesterol: 173mg

Scrambled Egg Pita Pocket

Prep time: 15 minutes | Cook time: 10 minutes

Eggs are a great option for breakfast because they supply a big punch of nutrients and are very filling. Eggs can be eaten a variety of ways—even in pita pockets!

Yield: 2 pita pockets

Serving size: 1 pita pocket

GLUTEN-FREE, NUT-FREE, SOY-FREE, VEGETARIAN, GOOD FOR PRE-CONCEPTION, KID-FRIENDLY, QUICK

1 tablespoon extra-virgin olive oil

1 cup cherry tomatoes, chopped

2 cups arugula

5 large eggs

Salt, for seasoning

Freshly ground black pepper, for seasoning

Feta cheese (optional; use pasteurized if you are currently pregnant)

2 pita pockets

Per serving: Calories: 381; Total fat: 19g; Saturated fat: 5g; Carbohydrate: 34g; Sugar: 4g; Fiber: 3g; Protein: 20g; Sodium: 472mg; Cholesterol: 409mg

1. Heat the oil in a medium sauté pan over medium-low heat.

2. Add the tomatoes to the pan and cook for 3 to 5 minutes.

3. Add the arugula to the pan and continue to cook for 1 minute more.

4. Meanwhile, crack the eggs into a bowl, season with salt and pepper, and whisk.

5. Add the eggs to the pan, mixing the veggies with the eggs until cooked, about 5 minutes.

6. Add the feta cheese, if using, and fill the two pita pockets with the scramble.

Tip: If you are having a hard time stomaching veggies (hello, first trimester), it's okay to leave them out. Avoid tomatoes and other highly acidic foods if you are experiencing heartburn.

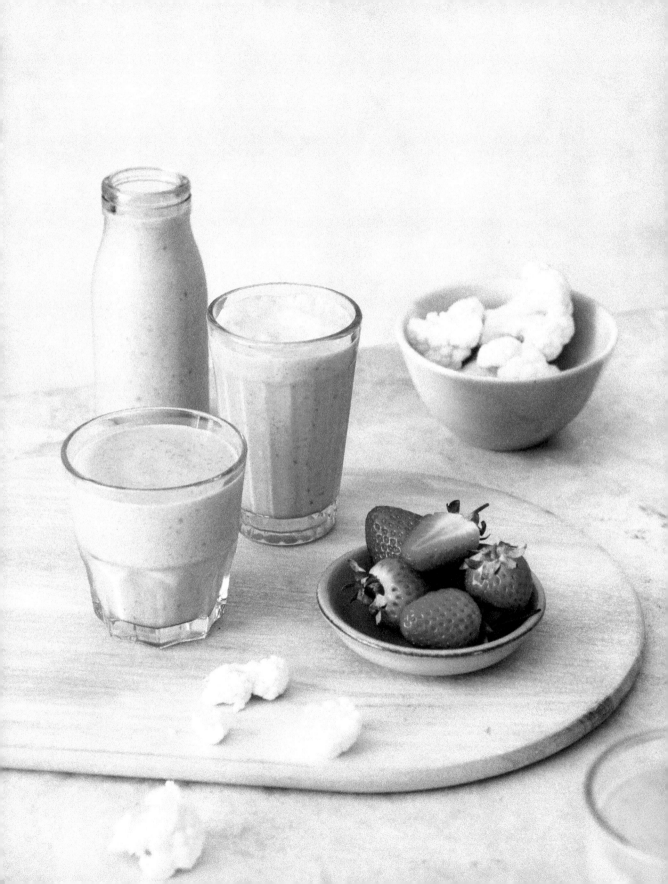

Protein-Packed Strawberry Smoothie

Prep time: 10 minutes

Smoothies are a good option if you are having a hard time eating full meals due to nausea, vomiting, or overall fatigue. They are effortless to consume and allow you to combine several food groups to maximize your nutrient intake.

Yield: 2 servings

Serving size: 1 cup

GLUTEN-FREE, NUT-FREE, SOY-FREE, VEGETARIAN, GOOD FOR NAUSEA, KID-FRIENDLY, QUICK

1 cup frozen strawberries
1 cup frozen cauliflower
2 tablespoons hemp seeds
1 cup full-fat, plain
   Greek yogurt
1 teaspoon maple syrup
   (optional)

Per serving: Calories: 263; Total fat: 18g; Saturated fat: 9g; Carbohydrate: 15g; Sugar: 12g; Fiber: 3g; Protein: 12g; Sodium: 129mg; Cholesterol: 0mg

Add all the ingredients to a blender and blend until the smoothie is the consistency you desire.

Tip: If you are used to supersweet smoothies, you may want to add a little maple syrup or another sweetener such as stevia.

Mango Carrot Smoothie

Prep time: 10 minutes

This smoothie tastes much better than V8 juice! Carrots are sweet, so they bring great flavor as well as nutrients to the smoothie.

Yield: 2 servings

Serving size: 1 cup

DAIRY-FREE, GLUTEN-FREE, SOY-FREE, VEGAN, GOOD FOR NAUSEA, GOOD FOR PRE-CONCEPTION, KID-FRIENDLY, QUICK

1 cup frozen mango
1 small banana
6 or 7 baby carrots
1 handful spinach
1 cup unsweetened
   almond milk
2 tablespoons almond butter

Per serving: Calories: 226; Total fat: 11g; Saturated fat: 1g; Carbohydrate: 31g; Sugar: 20g; Fiber: 6g; Protein: 6g; Sodium: 128mg; Cholesterol: 0mg

Add all the ingredients to a blender and blend until the smoothie is the consistency you desire.

Tip: The carrots have the potential to make the smoothie a bit chunky. Keep blending to make it smoother.

VEGGIE-FILLED OMELET

....

Prep time: 5 minutes | Cook time: 10 minutes

This omelet is a great breakfast for Saturday mornings. Experiment by adding various fillings such as artichokes, greens, and asparagus. A little creativity in the kitchen will prevent you from becoming bored with your meals.

....

Yield: 1 omelet

Serving size: 1 omelet

....

DAIRY-FREE, GLUTEN-FREE, NUT-FREE, SOY-FREE, VEGETARIAN, ENERGY ENHANCER, GESTATIONAL DIABETES–FRIENDLY, GOOD FOR CONSTIPATION, QUICK

....

1 tablespoon avocado oil

1 cup shredded kale

¾ cup sliced white mushrooms

3 large eggs

Salt, for seasoning

Freshly ground black pepper, for seasoning

Dried oregano, for seasoning

½ mini avocado or ¼ large avocado, pitted, peeled, and sliced (optional)

....

Per serving: Calories: 357; Total fat: 27g; Saturated fat: 6g; Carbohydrate: 10g; Sugar: 2g; Fiber: 2g; Protein: 20g; Sodium: 372mg; Cholesterol: 491mg

1. Heat the oil in a medium sauté pan over medium heat.

2. Add the kale and the mushrooms to the pan and sauté for 5 to 7 minutes, or until the kale is wilted.

3. In a medium bowl, whisk the eggs with the salt, pepper, and oregano.

4. Remove the veggies from pan and reduce the heat to medium-low.

5. Pour the eggs into the pan and move the pan around so the egg almost covers it. Cook the eggs until the edges begin to brown, about 3 minutes. Flip the omelet when there is almost no runny egg left on top and cook for 1 minute more.

6. Add the veggies to the omelet and fold it in half.

7. Remove the omelet from the pan and top it with avocado slices, if using.

Tip: Take this dish to the next level by topping the omelet with pesto from the Pesto Chicken Salad recipe (page 49)!

Kiwi, Cucumber, Kale Smoothie

Prep time: 10 minutes

This nourishing green smoothie is so refreshing. The chia seeds add fiber and important minerals such as calcium, magnesium, and zinc.

Yield: 2 servings

Serving size: 1 cup

DAIRY-FREE, GLUTEN-FREE, SOY-FREE, VEGAN, GOOD FOR LEG CRAMPS, MAY HELP WITH HEADACHES, QUICK

1 cup shredded kale
½ cup sliced cucumber
1 kiwi, peeled
1 cup water
2 tablespoons chia seeds
Juice of ½ lime

Add all the ingredients to a blender and blend until the smoothie is the consistency you desire.

Per serving: Calories: 125; Total fat: 5g; Saturated fat: 1g; Carbohydrate: 20g; Sugar: 5g; Fiber: 7g; Protein: 5g; Sodium: 20mg; Cholesterol: 0mg

Sweet Potato Muffins

Prep time: 15 minutes | Cook time: 30 to 40 minutes

These muffins are a little more involved than most of the other breakfasts in this book, but trust me—they are delicious! They taste like a dessert but contain no refined sugar.

Yield: 24 muffins

Serving size: 1 to 2 muffins

DAIRY-FREE, GLUTEN-FREE, SOY-FREE, VEGAN, GOOD FOR LACTATION, GOOD FOR LEG CRAMPS, GOOD FOR NAUSEA, KID-FRIENDLY

2 cups mashed sweet potato

1 ripe banana

2 tablespoons vanilla extract

1 tablespoon almond butter

⅓ cup maple syrup

1⅔ cups unsweetened almond milk

1 cup almond flour

1 cup gluten-free oats

1 teaspoon baking soda

1 teaspoon baking powder

1 tablespoon cinnamon

½ cup hemp hearts

Per serving: Calories: 207; Total fat: 8g; Saturated fat: 1g; Carbohydrate: 26g; Sugar: 9g; Fiber: 4g; Protein: 6g; Sodium: 190mg; Cholesterol: 0mg

1. Preheat the oven to 400°F.

2. In a large bowl, combine the sweet potatoes and the banana, beating with a hand mixer if there are still lumps.

3. Add the vanilla, almond butter, maple syrup, and almond milk to the sweet potatoes and banana. Stir to combine.

4. In a medium bowl, combine the flour, oats, baking soda, baking powder, cinnamon, and hemp hearts.

5. Mix the wet ingredients with the dry ingredients.

6. Line two muffin tins with 24 muffin cup liners and fill each cup two-thirds full with batter.

7. Bake for 30 minutes. If you are baking two pans at the same time, they may need to cook for 40 minutes.

Tip: These muffins are great to make if you are having sweet potatoes for dinner. Make one or two extra potatoes to mash for this recipe.

Edamame Frittata

Prep time: 20 minutes | Cook time: 15 minutes

No cookbook breakfast section is complete without a yummy frittata. This recipe is protein packed and simply delicious.

Yield: 4 servings

Serving size:
1 (2-inch) slice

NUT-FREE, VEGETARIAN, ENERGY ENHANCER, GOOD FOR POSTPARTUM RECOVERY, GOOD FOR PRE-CONCEPTION, QUICK

2 tablespoons extra-virgin olive oil
⅓ cup frozen shelled edamame
½ cup frozen corn
¼ cup chopped shallot
6 large eggs
1 teaspoon Italian seasoning
½ teaspoon salt
½ teaspoon freshly ground black pepper
¼ cup scallions, chopped
¼ cup goat cheese (pasteurized if you are currently pregnant)

1. Preheat the broiler.

2. Heat the oil in a large cast-iron skillet over medium-high heat and cook the edamame, corn, and shallot until the shallot is light brown, about 7 minutes.

3. Meanwhile, in a large bowl, whisk together the eggs, Italian seasoning, salt, and pepper. Add the scallions.

4. Pour the egg mixture into the skillet. Sprinkle on the cheese.

5. Transfer the skillet to the oven for 5 to 7 minutes, or until a kitchen thermometer shows the dish has reached an internal temperature of 165°F. You may have to shift the uncooked egg portion around the pan by lifting the pan up and turning it.

6. Move the skillet to within 6 inches of the heat source and broil for 1 minute. You may need to adjust the oven rack.

7. Once the top of the frittata is puffy and golden, remove it from the oven. Slice the frittata into wedges and enjoy.

Per serving: Calories: 213; Total fat: 16g; Saturated fat: 4g; Carbohydrate: 7g; Sugar: 2g; Fiber: 1g; Protein: 12g; Sodium: 416mg; Cholesterol: 250mg

CRUSTLESS SPINACH QUICHE

Prep time: 10 minutes | Cook time: 25 minutes

Quiche is so nice I've included it twice! This one is the easiest of the two recipes and is excellent if you are struggling with high blood sugar.

Yield: 6 servings

Serving size: 1 (2-inch) pie slice

GLUTEN-FREE, NUT-FREE, SOY-FREE, VEGETARIAN, GESTATIONAL DIABETES– FRIENDLY, QUICK

Coconut oil spray
1 tablespoon avocado oil
½ medium yellow onion, chopped
3 garlic cloves, minced
6 large eggs
Salt, for seasoning
Freshly ground black pepper, for seasoning
¼ cup heavy cream
1 cup mozzarella cheese
4 cups fresh spinach

1. Preheat the oven to 375°F. Spray a 9-inch pie plate with coconut oil.

2. Heat the avocado oil in a medium sauté pan over medium heat and cook the onion and the garlic until the onion begins to brown, 3 to 5 minutes.

3. Meanwhile, in a medium bowl, whisk together the eggs, salt, pepper, and heavy cream.

4. Stir in the cheese.

5. Place the veggies in the prepared pie plate and cover with the egg mixture.

6. Bake for 20 minutes or until the quiche begins to brown along the edges and a kitchen thermometer shows the dish has reached 160°F.

Per serving: Calories: 167; Total fat: 13g; Saturated fat: 6g; Carbohydrate: 3g; Sugar: 1g; Fiber: 1g; Protein: 11g; Sodium: 227mg; Cholesterol: 192mg

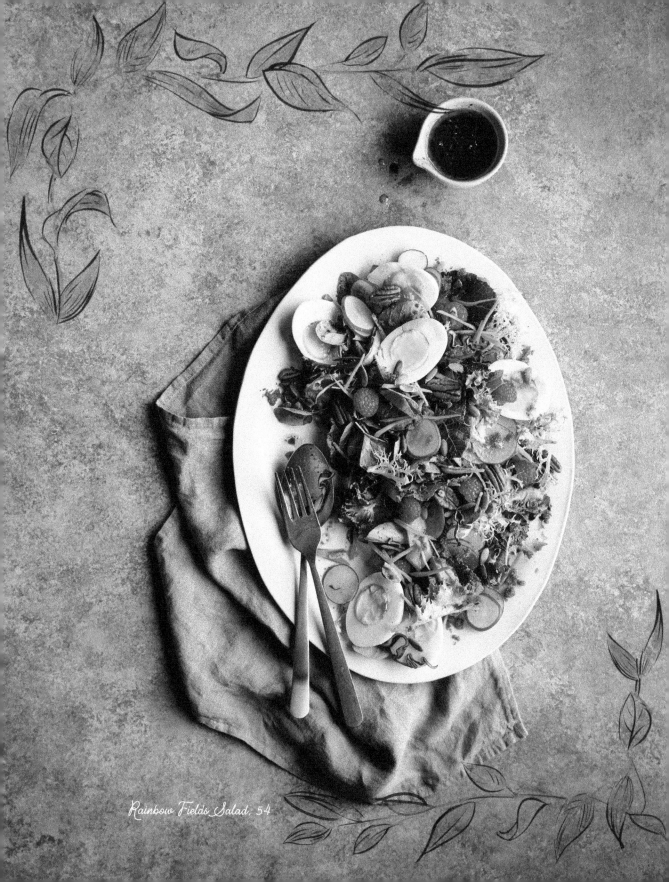

Rainbow Fields Salad, 54

CHAPTER FOUR

SALADS & SOUPS

Both salads and soups provide quick and delicious ways to add nutrient-rich vegetables and protein to your diet. You can also make soups during your last trimester of pregnancy to freeze and enjoy once the baby arrives.

CRAVE-WORTHY EGG SALAD

Prep time: 10 minutes

This recipe was created with the oh-so-common pickle craving in mind. The pickles add a savory salt and vinegar flavor. Be sure to include the egg yolks, which contain half the eggs' nutrients.

Yield: 4 servings

Serving size: ¾ cup

DAIRY-FREE, NUT-FREE, VEGETARIAN, GESTATIONAL DIABETES–FRIENDLY, GOOD FOR PRE-CONCEPTION, QUICK

6 hardboiled eggs, peeled and chopped

1 teaspoon finely chopped fresh dill

2 tablespoons chopped dill pickle or unsweetened relish

2 tablespoons mayonnaise

2 tablespoons mustard

Whole-wheat bread or lettuce wraps (optional, for serving)

Per serving: Calories: 170; Total fat: 13g; Saturated fat: 3g; Carbohydrate: 4g; Sugar: 1g; Fiber: 1g; Protein: 10g; Sodium: 434mg; Cholesterol: 248mg

1. In a medium bowl, combine the eggs, dill, pickle, mayonnaise, and mustard.

2. Mix all the ingredients together and enjoy the salad on its own, or on bread or lettuce wraps, if desired.

Tip: If you have gestational diabetes, eat the egg salad plain or with lettuce wraps to reduce your carb intake.

Stuffed Avocado Salmon Salad

Prep time: 10 minutes

Don't limit yourself to salmon fillets. Canned salmon provides the same amount of nutrients and requires much less prep work and cooking.

Yield: 4 servings

Serving size: 1 half of an avocado with ⅓ cup salmon salad

GLUTEN-FREE, NUT-FREE, SOY-FREE, GESTATIONAL DIABETES–FRIENDLY, GOOD FOR LACTATION, GOOD FOR LEG CRAMPS, MAY HELP WITH HEADACHES, QUICK

1 (6-ounce) can wild-caught salmon, drained

2 tablespoons mayonnaise

1 teaspoon lemon juice

½ teaspoon salt

½ teaspoon freshly ground black pepper

⅓ cup diced celery

⅓ cup diced red onion

2 medium avocados, halved and pitted

1. Place the salmon in a medium bowl.

2. Add the mayonnaise, lemon juice, salt, pepper, celery, and onion and stir to combine.

3. Add ⅓ cup of the salmon salad to each avocado half. If the holes left by the avocado pits are not big enough to hold the salad, use a spoon to hollow out the avocados a bit more.

Per serving: Calories: 251; Total fat: 20g; Saturated fat: 3g; Carbohydrate: 9g; Sugar: 1g; Fiber: 6g; Protein: 11g; Sodium: 510mg; Cholesterol: 15mg

Avocado Chicken Salad

Prep time: 10 minutes | Cook time: 30 minutes

My husband raves about this recipe. One week he insisted that I make it twice.

Yield: 4 servings

Serving size: 1 cup

DAIRY-FREE, GLUTEN-FREE, NUT-FREE, SOY-FREE, GESTATIONAL DIABETES–FRIENDLY, GOOD FOR LEG CRAMPS, GOOD FOR NAUSEA, GOOD FOR SWELLING

FOR THE CHICKEN
2 chicken breasts
Salt, for seasoning
Freshly ground black pepper, for seasoning

FOR THE SALAD
3 medium avocados, peeled, pitted, and cut into ¼-inch dice
2 tablespoons cilantro, finely chopped
2 tablespoons lime juice
Salt, for seasoning
Freshly ground black pepper, for seasoning
1 teaspoon chili powder (optional)
Tortilla chips or pita pockets (optional, for serving)

Per serving: Calories: 283; Total fat: 21g; Saturated fat: 3g; Carbohydrate: 12g; Sugar: 1g; Fiber: 9g; Protein: 15g; Sodium: 78mg; Cholesterol: 36mg

TO MAKE THE CHICKEN

1. Preheat the oven to 375°F.

2. Season the chicken on both sides with salt and pepper (or your other favorite seasoning).

3. Place the chicken on a baking sheet and bake for approximately 30 minutes. Use a kitchen thermometer to make sure the chicken reaches an internal temperature of 165°F. Alternatively, you can cook the chicken in a skillet on the stovetop over medium-high heat, again making sure to cook it to an internal temperature of 165°F.

TO MAKE THE SALAD

1. Shred or dice the cooked chicken breasts and place the meat in a large bowl. Add the avocado to the bowl.

2. Add the cilantro, lime juice, salt, pepper, and chili powder, if using.

3. Mix all the ingredients together.

4. Serve as is, with a handful of tortilla chips, or in a pita pocket, if desired.

> *Tip:* Because avocados brown easily, you'll want to eat this salad on the same day it is made.

Pesto Chicken Salad

Prep time: 10 minutes | Cook time: 5 minutes

This recipe makes a perfect workday lunch, and you can use the pesto sauce in many other dishes.

Yield: 4 servings
Serving size: 1 cup

GLUTEN-FREE, SOY-FREE, GESTATIONAL DIABETES–FRIENDLY, GOOD FOR POST-PARTUM RECOVERY, GOOD FOR PRE-CONCEPTION, KID-FRIENDLY, QUICK

⅓ cup extra-virgin olive oil plus 1 teaspoon, divided

1 red bell pepper, seeded and chopped

⅓ cup Parmesan cheese

¼ cup pine nuts

2 ounces fresh basil

Pinch salt

½ teaspoon freshly ground black pepper

Juice of ½ lemon

2 cups cooked and diced or shredded chicken (see Avocado Chicken Salad, page 48)

Per serving: Calories: 358; Total fat: 27g; Saturated fat: 5g; Carbohydrate: 5g; Sugar: 2g; Fiber: 1g; Protein: 26g; Sodium: 182mg; Cholesterol: 61mg

1. Heat 1 teaspoon of the oil in a small sauté pan over medium heat.

2. Add the bell pepper to the pan and cook for about 5 minutes.

3. In a food processor, combine the remaining ⅓ cup olive oil, the Parmesan cheese, pine nuts, basil, salt, pepper, and lemon juice. Blend until almost completely smooth.

4. Add the chicken and bell pepper to a medium bowl.

5. Add the pesto sauce to the bowl and mix everything together.

Tip: Instead of pine nuts, try making the pesto with walnuts or cashews!

BUTTER LETTUCE SALAD WITH SHRIMP

Prep time: 15 minutes

Butter lettuce has a soft, buttery texture (hence its name). Lettuce isn't as nutrient-dense as our good friends kale and spinach, but there's no harm in enjoying a variety of different greens.

Yield: 2 servings

Serving size: 2 cups

GLUTEN-FREE, SOY-FREE, GOOD FOR CONSTIPATION, GOOD FOR PRE-CONCEPTION, MAY HELP WITH HEADACHES, QUICK

FOR THE SALAD

4 cups chopped butter lettuce

¼ cup sliced red onion

¼ cup mandarin orange segments, unsweetened

¼ cup chopped walnuts

12 small to medium shrimp, cooked according to the Lemony Garlic Shrimp recipe (page 73)

FOR THE DRESSING

5 tablespoons extra-virgin olive oil

¼ cup apple cider vinegar

1 teaspoon Dijon mustard

2 teaspoons lemon juice

½ teaspoon salt

½ teaspoon freshly ground black pepper

1½ tablespoons maple syrup

Per serving: Calories: 540; Total fat: 46g; Saturated fat: 6g; Carbohydrate: 21g; Sugar: 15g; Fiber: 3g; Protein: 13g; Sodium: 847mg; Cholesterol: 145mg

TO MAKE THE SALAD

Place the lettuce in a large salad bowl and add the onion, orange, walnuts, and shrimp.

TO MAKE THE DRESSING

Whisk together all the dressing ingredients and add the dressing to the salad. Toss well to combine.

> *Tip:* The next time you make the Lemony Garlic Shrimp recipe (page 73) for dinner, use your leftovers to throw this salad together for a quick and delicious lunch the next day!

Kale and Quinoa Salad

Prep time: 10 minutes | Cook time: 15 minutes

Kale, as discussed on page 16, is really a superstar pregnancy green. This salad has the perfect mix of textures, incorporating crunchy chickpeas, almonds, and cucumbers as well as creamy avocado.

Yield: 2 servings

Serving size: 2 cups

DAIRY-FREE, GLUTEN-FREE, SOY-FREE, VEGAN, ENERGY ENHANCER, GESTATIONAL DIABETES–FRIENDLY, GOOD FOR CONSTIPATION, GOOD FOR PRE-CONCEPTION, MAY HELP WITH HEAD-ACHES, QUICK

FOR THE SALAD

½ cup uncooked quinoa, rinsed

4 cups chopped kale

½ cup blueberries

1 cup chopped cucumber

½ cup Roasted Chickpeas (page 114)

¼ cup almond slivers

2 tablespoons chia seeds

1 medium avocado, peeled, pitted, and chopped

FOR THE DRESSING

¼ cup extra-virgin olive oil

¼ cup lemon juice

1 tablespoon honey

1½ teaspoons Dijon mustard

¼ teaspoon salt

Pinch freshly ground black pepper

TO MAKE THE SALAD

1. Place the quinoa in a small pot with 1 cup of water and bring it to a boil over high heat. Reduce the heat to low, cover, and let it simmer for 15 minutes. When all the water has been absorbed, fluff the quinoa with a fork.

2. Combine the quinoa in a large bowl with the kale, blueberries, cucumber, chickpeas, almonds, chia seeds, and avocado.

TO MAKE THE DRESSING

Whisk together all the dressing ingredients and add the dressing to the salad. Toss well to combine.

Per serving: Calories: 863; Total fat: 52g; Saturated fat: 7g; Carbohydrate: 86g; Sugar: 15g; Fiber: 18g; Protein: 21g; Sodium: 503mg; Cholesterol: 0mg

Tip: Use your hands to massage the kale with a little bit of lemon juice and olive oil for 2 to 3 minutes before adding it to the other ingredients. This will soften the leaves and make them more palatable.

Rustic Italian Salad

Prep time: 15 minutes

This recipe is my attempt to recreate one of my favorite Trader Joe's salads. It's simple, fresh, and full of satisfying Mediterranean flavors.

Yield: 2 servings

Serving size: 2 cups

GLUTEN-FREE, NUT-FREE, SOY-FREE, GOOD FOR CONSTIPATION, QUICK

FOR THE SALAD

4 cups chopped romaine lettuce

1½ cups cooked and diced chicken (see Avocado Chicken Salad, page 48)

1 cup chopped cherry tomatoes

2 carrots, chopped

1 green bell pepper, seeded and chopped

1 (15-ounce) can white beans, drained and rinsed

½ cup grated Parmesan cheese

FOR THE DRESSING

¼ cup extra-virgin olive oil

2 tablespoons lemon juice

1½ teaspoons Dijon mustard

2 tablespoons red wine vinegar

1 teaspoon oregano

¼ teaspoon salt

Pinch freshly ground black pepper

TO MAKE THE SALAD

In a large bowl, combine the lettuce, chicken, tomatoes, carrots, bell pepper, beans, and Parmesan cheese.

TO MAKE THE DRESSING

Whisk together the dressing ingredients and add the dressing to the salad. Toss well to combine.

Per serving: Calories: 584; Total fat: 33g; Saturated fat: 8g; Carbohydrate: 39g; Sugar: 9g; Fiber: 9g; Protein: 40g; Sodium: 684mg; Cholesterol: 65mg

Taco Jar Salad

Prep time: 20 minutes | Cook time: 10 minutes

Layering a colorful salad in a mason jar is a practical and fun way to prepare an easy-to-transport lunch for work. Store the dressing and crunchy chips separately and add them right before you eat the salad.

Yield: 2 servings

Serving size: 2 cups

GLUTEN-FREE, SOY-FREE, ENERGY ENHANCER, GOOD FOR CONSTIPATION, GOOD FOR PRE-CONCEPTION, GOOD FOR SWELLING, KID-FRIENDLY

FOR THE SALAD

1½ cups ground beef

2 teaspoons chili powder

1 teaspoon cumin

4 cups chopped green leaf lettuce

1 (15-ounce) can corn, rinsed and drained

1 (15-ounce) can black beans, rinsed and drained

½ cup chopped tomatoes

½ cup Mexican cheese blend

2 tablespoons chopped fresh cilantro

½ cup corn tortilla chips, crushed

FOR THE DRESSING

1 medium avocado, peeled and pitted

¼ cup cilantro

Juice of ½ lime

¼ cup sour cream

¼ cup water

¼ teaspoon salt

Pinch chili powder

TO MAKE THE SALAD

1. In a large skillet over medium heat, cook the ground beef with the chili powder and cumin until browned and fully cooked, about 10 minutes.

2. In a 16-ounce mason jar, layer lettuce, beef, corn, beans, and tomatoes.

3. Add cheese and cilantro to the top of the salad. Store the crushed tortilla chips in a separate container and add right before eating.

TO MAKE THE DRESSING

Add all the dressing ingredients to a blender or food processor and blend well. Drizzle the dressing into the jar just prior to serving.

Per serving: Calories: 888; Total fat: 44g; Saturated fat: 16g; Carbohydrate: 90g; Sugar: 6g; Fiber: 29g; Protein: 43g; Sodium: 689mg; Cholesterol: 75mg

Rainbow Fields Salad

Prep time: 20 minutes | Cook time: 20 to 25 minutes

This salad has it all! A rainbow of beautiful fruits and veggies make it bright and nutritious.

Yield: 2 servings

Serving size: 2 cups

DAIRY-FREE, GLUTEN-FREE,
SOY-FREE, VEGETARIAN,
GOOD FOR CONSTIPATION,
GOOD FOR LACTATION

½ cup uncooked teff

4 cups chopped leafy greens

½ cup sliced radish

1 cup raspberries

½ cup shredded carrot

1 yellow bell pepper, seeded
   and diced

1 cup chopped
   purple cabbage

¼ cup pecans

¼ cup pumpkin seeds

3 hardboiled eggs, peeled
   and chopped

¼ cup Simple Go-To Salad
   Dressing (page 150)

Per serving: Calories: 587;
Total fat: 42g; Saturated fat:
8g; Carbohydrate: 39g; Sugar:
11g; Fiber: 12g; Protein: 20g;
Sodium: 266mg; Cholesterol:
248mg

1. In a medium pot, bring the teff and 2 cups of water to a boil. Reduce heat to low, cover, and let it simmer for 15 to 20 minutes.

2. Allow the teff to cool for at least 5 minutes before adding it to the salad.

3. In a large bowl, mix together the greens, radish, raspberries, carrot, bell pepper, and cabbage. Add the pecans and pumpkin seeds.

4. Toss the salad with the dressing and top with the eggs before serving.

Tip: Teff is similar to quinoa in that it is actually a seed and is gluten-free. It is a decent source of calcium and tops the charts in manganese.

Wild Arugula, Spinach, and Steak Salad

Prep time: 20 minutes, plus 1 hour or overnight to marinate | Cook time: 25 minutes

This is one of my favorite salads! I especially love the combination of flavors and nutrients it provides.

Yield: 2 to 3 servings

Serving size: 2 cups

GLUTEN-FREE, SOY-FREE, ENERGY ENHANCER, GESTATIONAL DIABETES–FRIENDLY, GOOD FOR CONSTIPATION, GOOD FOR PRE-CONCEPTION

FOR THE MARINADE

1 tablespoon minced garlic
¼ cup lemon juice
¼ cup balsamic vinegar
¼ cup extra-virgin olive oil

FOR THE SALAD

1 pound flank steak
2 cups spinach
2 cups arugula
1 cup sliced strawberries
¼ cup walnuts
¼ cup Gorgonzola cheese
   (pasteurized if you are
   currently pregnant)
1 medium avocado, peeled,
   pitted, and diced

FOR THE DRESSING

¼ cup extra-virgin olive oil
2 tablespoons
   balsamic vinegar
1 tablespoon honey
1 teaspoon Dijon mustard
¼ teaspoon salt
¼ teaspoon freshly ground
   black pepper

TO MAKE THE STEAK

1. In a small bowl, whisk together the marinade ingredients. Transfer the marinade to a bag or shallow pan and place the steak in the marinade so it is covered as much as possible. Let the steak marinate in the refrigerator for at least one hour or overnight.

2. Cook the steak in a large cast-iron skillet over medium heat, about 20 minutes, or until a kitchen thermometer shows it has reached an internal temperature of 165°F.

TO MAKE THE SALAD

1. In a large bowl, combine the spinach, arugula, strawberries, walnuts, cheese, and avocado.

2. Once the steak has finished cooking and rested for 5 minutes, slice it thinly, and add it to the salad.

TO MAKE THE DRESSING

In a small bowl, whisk together the dressing ingredients. Drizzle the dressing over the salad just prior to serving.

Per serving: Calories: 723; Total fat: 53g; Saturated fat: 14g; Carbohydrate: 19g; Sugar: 9g; Fiber: 7g; Protein: 48g; Sodium: 542mg; Cholesterol: 121mg

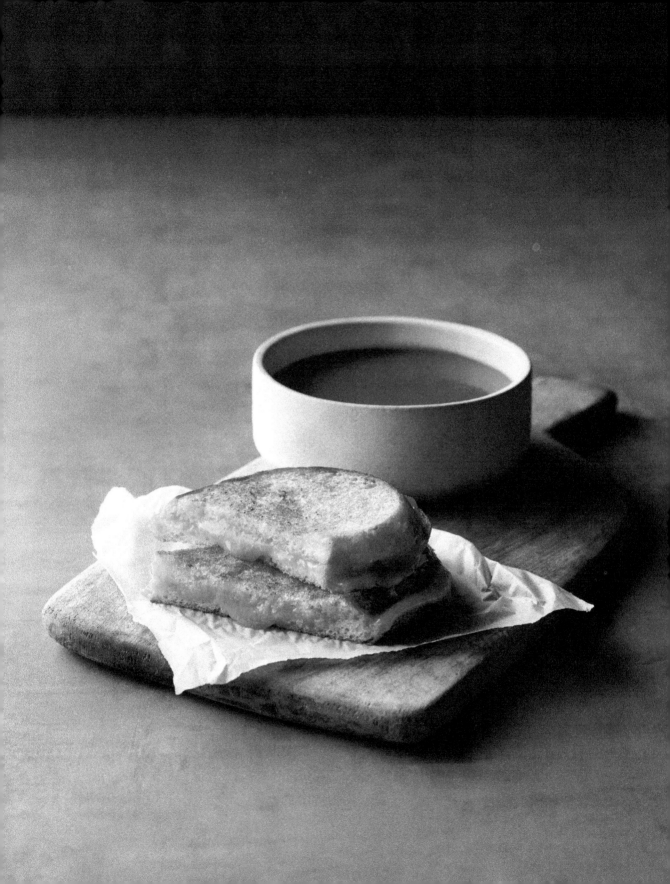

CLASSIC TOMATO SOUP AND GRILLED CHEESE

Prep time: 15 minutes | Cook time: 1 hour and 35 minutes

You can make tomato soup using canned tomatoes, but this soup is much tastier because you roast fresh tomatoes yourself. It's the perfect accompaniment to a toasty grilled cheese sandwich.

Yield: 6 to 8 servings

Serving size: 1 cup

NUT-FREE, SOY-FREE, VEGETARIAN, GOOD FOR LEG CRAMPS, GOOD FOR NAUSEA, GOOD FOR POSTPARTUM RECOVERY, KID-FRIENDLY

FOR THE SOUP

10 plum tomatoes, halved
2 tablespoons plus
   2 teaspoons extra-virgin
   olive oil, divided
1 teaspoon salt
1½ teaspoons freshly ground
   black pepper
2 medium yellow
   onions, chopped
4 garlic cloves, minced
¼ teaspoon red pepper flakes
1 (28-ounce) can plum
   tomatoes, with their juices
6 fresh basil leaves, chopped
1 teaspoon chopped
   fresh thyme
1 quart vegetable stock

FOR THE SANDWICHES

1 loaf sourdough bread
2 tablespoons butter
1 package Cheddar cheese
   deli slices

TO MAKE THE SOUP

1. Preheat the oven to 400°F.

2. In a large bowl, toss the fresh tomatoes in 2 tablespoons of oil, the salt, and pepper.

3. Spread out the tomatoes in one even layer on a rimmed baking sheet and roast for 40 to 45 minutes.

4. Heat the remaining 2 teaspoons of oil in an 8-quart stockpot over medium heat and sauté the onions, garlic, and red pepper flakes for 10 minutes, or until the onions start to turn brown.

5. Add the canned tomatoes, basil, thyme, and vegetable stock.

6. Add the oven-roasted tomatoes, including the juices on the baking sheet.

7. Bring the soup to a boil and simmer, uncovered, for 40 minutes.

8. Use an immersion blender to combine all of the ingredients or transfer the soup to a blender.

9. Taste the soup and add additional salt and pepper as needed. Serve hot or cold.

CONTINUED

TO MAKE THE SANDWICHES

1. Cut one slice of bread in half.

2. Butter one side of each half of the bread.

3. Heat a small skillet over medium heat.

4. Place one slice of bread in the skillet, buttered-side down.

5. Cut a slice of cheese in half and place it on top of the slice of bread in the skillet. Add the second slice of bread to the top, buttered-side up.

6. Cook for 1 minute on each side, or until both sides are golden brown and the cheese is melted.

7. Repeat steps 1 to 6 to make additional sandwiches.

Per serving: Calories: 509; Total fat: 28g; Saturated fat: 15g; Carbohydrate: 54g; Sugar: 13g; Fiber: 6g; Protein: 20g; Sodium: 1864mg; Cholesterol: 52mg

Warm Lentil and Kale Soup

Prep time: 10 minutes | Cook time: 45 minutes

This soup will warm and nourish your soul. It can be stored in the freezer for three to four months, so it is perfect to make before your baby arrives!

Yield: 6 servings

Serving size: 1 cup

DAIRY-FREE, GLUTEN-FREE, NUT-FREE, SOY-FREE, GOOD FOR CONSTIPATION, GOOD FOR POSTPARTUM RECOVERY, GOOD FOR PRE-CONCEPTION

1 tablespoon extra-virgin olive oil

1 cup chopped celery

1 cup chopped carrots

1 cup chopped onion

1 tablespoon minced garlic

1 teaspoon cumin

1 teaspoon thyme

1 teaspoon turmeric

1 teaspoon salt

1 teaspoon freshly ground black pepper

1 cup dry whole green lentils

4 cups (32 ounces) vegetable broth

3 scoops collagen peptide powder (optional; omit if vegetarian—adds extra protein and the amino acid glycine)

3 large handfuls kale, torn into bite-size pieces

1 cup white mushrooms, sliced

Per serving: Calories: 173; Total fat: 3g; Saturated fat: 0g; Carbohydrate: 29g; Sugar: 4g; Fiber: 7g; Protein: 9g; Sodium: 787mg; Cholesterol: 0mg

1. Heat the oil in a large stockpot over medium heat and sauté the celery, carrots, onion, garlic, cumin, thyme, turmeric, salt, and pepper, stirring occasionally, for about 5 minutes, or until the veggies are slightly tender.

2. Add the lentils and broth. Also add the collagen powder, if using. Increase the heat to high and let it come to a boil.

3. Reduce the heat to low and cover. Let the soup simmer for 35 to 40 minutes, or until the lentils are tender.

4. Add the kale and mushrooms and cook for 3 to 5 minutes, or until they become tender. Serve warm.

Tip: To make this recipe in an Instant Pot®, after adding the lentils and broth in step 2, select the soup/broth setting, and set the timer for 10 minutes. Make sure the lid is set to the sealed position before starting the timer. Quick release the pressure and open the lid to add the mushrooms and kale. Select the sauté setting and stir the soup until the veggies become tender, 3 to 5 minutes.

Easy Chicken Chili

Prep time: 10 minutes | Cook time: 25 minutes

I can't believe how easy and tasty this chili is! It's fantastic for a lazy week-night dinner when all you want to do it is throw a bunch of ingredients in a pot and eat.

Yield: 6 servings
Serving size: 1 cup

GLUTEN-FREE, NUT-FREE, SOY-FREE, GOOD FOR LEG CRAMPS, GOOD FOR NAUSEA, GOOD FOR POST-PARTUM RECOVERY, QUICK

1 teaspoon avocado oil
½ medium yellow onion, chopped
4 garlic cloves, minced
1 pound boneless chicken, diced
16 ounces chicken broth
¼ cup whole milk
1 can white beans
1 (15-ounce) can whole kernel corn (not sweet)
2 (4.5-ounce) cans green chiles
1 teaspoon oregano
1 teaspoon cumin
1 teaspoon paprika

Per serving: Calories: 219; Total fat: 4g; Saturated fat: 1g; Carbohydrate: 21g; Sugar: 3g; Fiber: 4g; Protein: 21g; Sodium: 475mg; Cholesterol: 49mg

1. Heat the oil in a large stockpot over medium heat and sauté the onion and garlic for 3 to 5 minutes.

2. Add the chicken and cook for about 10 minutes, or until it is cooked all the way through.

3. Add the broth, milk, beans, corn, chiles, oregano, cumin, and paprika.

4. Let the soup simmer on medium-low heat for 10 minutes.

Tip: For even faster prep, buy precooked chicken and skip the cooking in step 2.

Chicken and Wild Rice Soup

Prep time: 10 minutes | Cook time: 1 hour

This is one of my go-to soups, especially because it can also be made in a slow cooker or Instant Pot®. The veggies provide a bit of crunch while the classic combination of rice, chicken, and mushrooms adds sustenance.

Yield: 6 servings
Serving size: 1 cup

GLUTEN-FREE, NUT-FREE, SOY-FREE, ENERGY ENHANCER, GOOD FOR POSTPARTUM RECOVERY

1 teaspoon avocado oil
1 cup chopped onion
1 tablespoon minced garlic
1 pound boneless chicken, cut into 1½-inch pieces
1 cup chopped celery
1 cup chopped carrots
4 cups (32 ounces) chicken broth
½ cup uncooked wild rice
2 cups heavy cream
4 ounces cream cheese
2 cups sliced cremini mushrooms
2 teaspoons dried thyme
2 teaspoons salt
1 teaspoon freshly ground black pepper

Per serving: Calories: 531; Total fat: 40g; Saturated fat: 23g; Carbohydrate: 19g; Sugar: 3g; Fiber: 2g; Protein: 25g; Sodium: 910mg; Cholesterol: 177mg

1. Heat the oil in a large stockpot over medium heat. Add the onion and garlic and sauté for 3 to 5 minutes.

2. Add the chicken and sauté for about 10 minutes, or until cooked through.

3. Add the celery and carrots and sauté for 2 more minutes.

4. Add the broth, rice, heavy cream, and cream cheese, stirring to combine.

5. Turn the heat up to high and bring the soup to a boil. Reduce the heat to low, cover, and let the soup simmer for 30 minutes.

6. Add the mushrooms, thyme, salt, and pepper and simmer for an additional 10 minutes, or until the mushrooms are tender.

Tip: For faster prep, use a rotisserie chicken and mirepoix (a pre-cut mix of celery, carrots, and onion).

Broccoli Cream Soup

Prep time: 10 minutes | Cook time: 20 minutes

Broccoli is an underrated cruciferous vegetable. A great source of vitamins C and K as well as potassium, it also adds some folate and protein to this soup.

Yield: 6 servings
Serving size: 1 cup

GLUTEN-FREE, NUT-FREE,
SOY-FREE, VEGETARIAN,
GOOD FOR POSTPARTUM
RECOVERY, KID-FRIENDLY

1 teaspoon avocado oil
½ medium yellow
　onion, chopped
3 garlic cloves, minced
2 cups (16 ounces)
　vegetable broth
½ cup heavy cream
2 cups Cheddar cheese
½ cup plain whole milk yogurt
4 cups fresh broccoli florets
1 teaspoon salt
1 teaspoon freshly ground
　black pepper

1. Heat the oil in a large stockpot over medium heat. Add the onion and garlic and sauté for 3 to 5 minutes.

2. Add the broth, heavy cream, cheese, and yogurt.

3. Add the broccoli and lower the heat to medium-low, cooking the broccoli until it's tender, about 10 minutes. Add the salt and pepper.

4. Use an immersion blender or place the soup in a food processor and blend until smooth.

Per serving: Calories: 279; Total fat: 22g; Saturated fat: 13g; Carbohydrate: 8g; Sugar: 3g; Fiber: 2g; Protein: 14g; Sodium: 900mg; Cholesterol: 69mg

Delicata Squash Soup

Prep time: 15 minutes | Cook time: 35 minutes

Delicata squash adds sweetness as well as nutrients, including fiber, magnesium, manganese, and vitamins C and B, to this soup. Its peel is edible, so there's no need to remove it.

Yield: 2 to 3 servings

Serving size: 1 cup

DAIRY-FREE, GLUTEN-FREE, NUT-FREE, SOY-FREE, VEGAN, GOOD FOR LEG CRAMPS, GOOD FOR POST-PARTUM RECOVERY

1 delicata squash, halved and seeded (seeds reserved)

3 tablespoons extra-virgin olive oil, divided

Salt, for seasoning

Freshly ground black pepper, for seasoning

1 teaspoon turmeric

1 medium yellow onion, chopped

3 garlic cloves, minced

1 cup vegetable broth

Per serving: Calories: 297; Total fat: 22g; Saturated fat: 3g; Carbohydrate: 9g; Sugar: 8g; Fiber: 1g; Protein: 6g; Sodium: 1712mg; Cholesterol: 0mg

1. Preheat the oven to 400°F.

2. Place the squash on a baking sheet, cut-side up. Drizzle 1 tablespoon of oil over the squash, and season both halves with the salt and pepper. Roast for 30 minutes.

3. Toss the squash seeds with 1 tablespoon of olive oil, salt, pepper, and turmeric. Place on a separate baking sheet and roast for 15 to 20 minutes.

4. Heat the remaining tablespoon of oil in a medium sauté pan over medium heat. Add three-fourths of the chopped onion and sauté for 2 minutes. Add the garlic and cook for another minute. Transfer the onion and garlic to a small bowl and set aside.

5. Add the remaining one-fourth of the onion to the pan and sauté until translucent, about 3 minutes. Remove from the heat.

CONTINUED

6. When the squash is done roasting, let it cool for a few minutes before chopping it into 2-inch pieces.

7. Add the squash, three-fourths of the onion, garlic, and broth to a blender. Blend until smooth.

8. Top the soup with the remaining sautéed onions and roasted squash seeds.

> *Tip:* Make a double batch of this soup and freeze it for up to 4 months. Thaw it overnight in the refrigerator before reheating.

CREAMY POTATO SOUP

Prep time: 15 minutes | Cook time: 25 minutes

If you are looking for a filling and satisfying soup, this is it! Potatoes are rich in potassium and a good source of fiber, magnesium, and vitamin C.

Yield: 6 servings
Serving size: 1 cup

GLUTEN-FREE, NUT-FREE, SOY-FREE, GOOD FOR NAUSEA, GOOD FOR POSTPARTUM RECOVERY, KID-FRIENDLY

6 uncooked bacon slices, diced
1 small yellow onion, diced
3 garlic cloves, minced
3 tablespoons flour
5 cups chicken broth
1 cup whole milk
1 cup half-and-half
3 pounds of gold potatoes, peeled and cut into 1-inch dice
1½ teaspoons salt
¼ teaspoon freshly ground black pepper
¼ cup sour cream
1 cup shredded sharp Cheddar cheese
Diced scallion, chopped bacon, and extra cheese (for topping; optional)

Per serving: Calories: 480; Total fat: 23g; Saturated fat: 12g; Carbohydrate: 46g; Sugar: 6g; Fiber: 7g; Protein: 22g; Sodium: 1812mg; Cholesterol: 64mg

1. In an eight-quart pot, cook the bacon over medium heat until crisp. Transfer the bacon to a paper towel–lined plate to drain. Leave the bacon fat in the pot.

2. Add the onion to the pot to cook until soft and translucent, 5 to 6 minutes. Add the garlic and cook 1 minute.

3. Stir in the flour until a paste forms. Cook for 2 to 3 minutes, or until it is a light golden color.

4. Pour in the broth, milk, and half-and-half. Add the potatoes, salt, and pepper. Stir to combine.

5. Bring the soup to a boil and then let it simmer, stirring occasionally, until the potatoes are softened and easily mashed, about 15 minutes.

6. Turn off the heat and use an immersion blender to purée the soup until most of the potatoes are smooth and creamy. You can also use a blender or food processor for this step.

7. With the heat off, stir in the sour cream and cheese. Add the bacon to the soup and stir to combine. Serve with diced scallion, chopped bacon, and extra cheese, if desired.

Tip: To make this soup vegetarian, use vegetable broth and eliminate the bacon.

Simple Veggie Soup

Prep time: 20 minutes | Cook time: 25 minutes

Who doesn't need a classic vegetable medley soup in their repertoire? If you are feeling under the weather or just looking for something comforting, this recipe should do the trick.

Yield: 8 to 10 servings
Serving size: 1 to 2 cups

DAIRY-FREE, GLUTEN-FREE, NUT-FREE, SOY-FREE, VEGAN, GESTATIONAL DIABETES–FRIENDLY, GOOD FOR NAUSEA, KID-FRIENDLY

1 tablespoon extra-virgin olive oil
1 medium yellow onion, chopped
4 garlic cloves, minced
4 cups vegetable broth
2 sweet potatoes, diced
4 medium carrots, chopped
Salt, for seasoning
Freshly ground black pepper, for seasoning
1 yellow squash, sliced
1 green zucchini, sliced
1 yellow bell pepper, seeded and chopped
1 red bell pepper, seeded and chopped
1 cup canned kidney beans, rinsed

Per serving: Calories: 128; Total fat: 3g; Saturated fat: 1g; Carbohydrate: 21g; Sugar: 6g; Fiber: 5g; Protein: 6g; Sodium: 510mg; Cholesterol: 0mg

1. Heat the oil in a large stockpot over medium heat. Add the onion and sauté for 3 to 5 minutes. Add the garlic and sauté for 1 minute.

2. Add the broth and bring to a boil. Add the sweet potatoes and carrots and season with salt and pepper. Lower the heat to medium and cook for 10 minutes.

3. Add the squash, zucchini, and bell peppers, stirring to combine.

4. Last, add in the beans, heat until warmed through, about 10 minutes, and serve.

Tip: If you are not vegan or vegetarian, try using bone broth instead of vegetable broth. Also feel free to be creative with the type of beans you use—try red, black, white, or navy.

SECRET INGREDIENT BEEF CHILI

Prep time: 20 minutes | Cook time: 40 minutes

This hearty chili is great to eat during postpartum recovery. Its potassium, sodium, and magnesium can help relieve leg cramps during pregnancy. If you are struggling with heartburn, you may want to skip this tomato-based meal.

Yield: 6 servings
Serving size: 1 cup

DAIRY-FREE, NUT-FREE, SOY-FREE, GOOD FOR LEG CRAMPS, GOOD FOR POSTPARTUM RECOVERY, KID-FRIENDLY

1 tablespoon extra-virgin olive oil

1 medium yellow onion, chopped

4 garlic cloves, minced

8 ounces grass-fed ground beef

2 (14-ounce) cans tomato sauce

1 (14-ounce) can crushed tomatoes

3 cups canned black beans, drained and rinsed

2½ tablespoons chili powder

1 teaspoon cocoa powder (secret ingredient)

½ teaspoon salt

1 teaspoon red pepper flakes (optional)

Per serving: Calories: 279; Total fat: 7g; Saturated fat: 2g; Carbohydrate: 37g; Sugar: 10g; Fiber: 13g; Protein: 19g; Sodium: 1073mg; Cholesterol: 26mg

1. Heat the oil in a large stockpot over medium heat. Add the onion and sauté for 3 to 5 minutes. Add the garlic and sauté for an additional minute.

2. Add the ground beef and cook until the meat is no longer pink.

3. Add the tomato sauce, tomatoes, beans, chili powder, cocoa powder, salt, and pepper.

4. Reduce the heat to medium-low and simmer for 30 minutes.

Tip: This recipe is usually made with 1 (12-ounce) bottle of beer, which is added after the beef is cooked. It adds more depth of the flavor, so I would recommend trying it! The longer you cook the chili, the more the alcohol cooks off, so if you do decide to add the beer, simmer the chili for at least 30 minutes.

TOFU MISO SOUP

Prep time: 30 minutes | Cook time: 30 minutes

This recipe is a take on ramen with a few fancy twists. It features the savory flavor of miso, a Japanese fermented soybean paste that provides probiotics.

Yield: 2 to 3 servings

Serving size: 1 cup

DAIRY-FREE, NUT-FREE, GOOD FOR LEG CRAMPS, GOOD FOR POSTPARTUM RECOVERY

7 ounces extra firm tofu
½ cup soy sauce
1 tablespoon garlic powder
1 teaspoon extra-virgin olive oil
3 garlic cloves, minced
2 tablespoons white miso paste
2 tablespoons hot water
Salt, for seasoning
4 to 6 ounces Udon or soba noodles
3 cups vegetable broth
1 teaspoon grated fresh ginger
1 teaspoon sesame oil
1 bunch (3 ounces) bok choy
Black sesame seeds and chopped scallions (for garnish; optional)

1. Preheat oven to 400°F and line a baking sheet with parchment paper. Set aside.

2. Drain the tofu and cut it in half lengthwise. Use a paper towel to absorb any extra moisture from the tofu and then cut it into 1-inch squares.

3. In a small bowl, combine the soy sauce and garlic powder. Coat the tofu in the soy sauce mixture.

4. Place the tofu on the prepared baking sheet and roast it in the oven for 15 minutes or until golden brown.

5. Heat the oil in a medium pot over medium heat. Add the garlic and cook for 1 minute.

6. Fill a second medium pot with water and bring to a boil over high heat.

7. In a small bowl, whisk the miso paste with the hot water. Add it to the first pot with the garlic.

8. Once the water in the second pot is boiling, season it with salt and add the noodles.

9. Add the broth to the first pot with the garlic and miso paste. Then add the ginger and sesame oil.

10. Turn the first pot down to medium-low and add the bok choy. Cook until it becomes tender, about 10 minutes.

11. Drain the noodles from the second pot and add them to the broth in the first pot.

12. Remove the tofu from the oven, add it to the broth, or wait and add it to individual bowls.

13. Garnish with black sesame seeds and scallions, if desired.

Per serving: Calories: 481; Total fat: 15g; Saturated fat: 2g; Carbohydrate: 56g; Sugar: 9g; Fiber: 5g; Protein: 33g; Sodium: 324mg; Cholesterol: 0mg

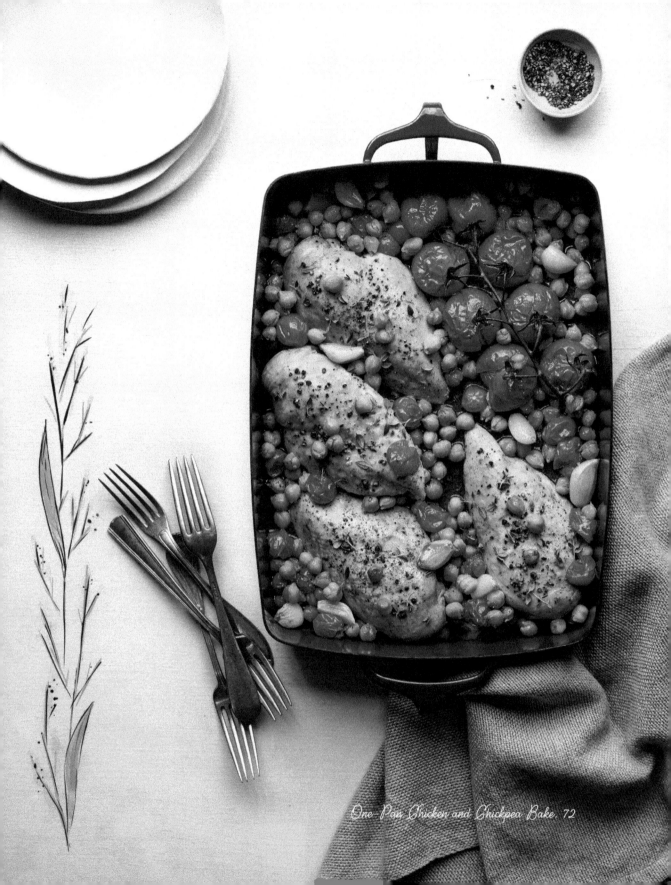

One-Pan Chicken and Chickpea Bake, 72

CHAPTER FIVE

MAIN DISHES

Main dishes are often associated with dinnertime, but the recipes in this chapter could work well for lunch, too. When you are tired and hungry during or after a long day, you'll find these recipes quick and easy to make. They'll also add variety to your weekly meal routine.

ONE-PAN CHICKEN AND CHICKPEA BAKE

Prep time: 10 minutes | Cook time: 30 minutes

One-pan dinners are great for busy weeknights. Preheat the oven, add everything to the pan, bake for a bit, and dinner is ready.

Yield: 4 servings

Serving size:

1 (3- to 4-ounce) chicken breast with ¾ cup chickpeas and tomatoes

DAIRY-FREE, GLUTEN-FREE, NUT-FREE, SOY-FREE, GESTATIONAL DIABETES–FRIENDLY, GREAT FOR POSTPARTUM RECOVERY

Coconut oil spray or olive oil spray
4 boneless chicken breasts
½ teaspoon salt
½ teaspoon freshly ground black pepper
1 (15.5-ounce) can chickpeas, drained and rinsed
1 cup cherry tomatoes
10 garlic cloves, minced (if you aren't a big garlic fan, use 5)
6 to 8 tomatoes on the vine
2 to 3 sprigs of thyme

1. Preheat the oven to 375°F. Spray a baking sheet with oil.

2. Season the chicken breasts with salt and pepper and place them on the pan.

3. Wash the cherry tomatoes and tomatoes on the vine.

4. Scatter the chickpeas, cherry tomatoes, and garlic around the chicken as evenly as possible, placing some garlic on top of the chicken breasts to allow the garlic flavor to soak in. Place the tomatoes on the vine directly on the baking sheet with the rest of the ingredients.

5. Bake for 30 minutes or until the chicken is cooked all the way through and a kitchen thermometer shows it has reached an internal temperature of 165°F.

6. Run your fingers down the thyme to break the leaves off and sprinkle them on top of the chicken bake after cooking for a pretty and flavorful garnish.

Per serving: Calories: 278; Total fat: 4g; Saturated fat: 0g; Carbohydrate: 29g; Sugar: 1g; Fiber: 6g; Protein: 30g; Sodium: 680mg; Cholesterol: 72mg

LEMONY GARLIC SHRIMP

Prep time: 10 minutes, plus 30 to 60 minutes to marinate
Cook time: 10 to 15 minutes

Shrimp are a good seafood option during pregnancy because they are relatively small, which means they contain relatively less mercury. Shrimp also provide selenium, vitamin B12, and DHA. To eliminate any health concerns, ensure that they are adequately cooked before you eat them.

Yield: 2 servings
Serving size: 6 shrimp

DAIRY-FREE, GLUTEN-FREE, NUT-FREE, SOY-FREE, GESTATIONAL DIABETES– FRIENDLY, GOOD FOR PRE-CONCEPTION, MAY HELP WITH HEADACHES

2 tablespoons minced garlic
Juice of ½ large lemon
1 tablespoon extra-virgin olive oil
½ teaspoon salt
12 medium to large frozen, uncooked shrimp*

Per serving: Calories; 244; Total fat: 9g; Saturated fat: 2g; Carbohydrate: 3g; Sugar: 0g; Fiber: 0g; Protein: 36g; Sodium: 966mg; Cholesterol: 332mg

1. In a medium mixing bowl, combine the garlic, lemon juice, oil, and salt.

2. Add the shrimp to the bowl to marinate in the mixture. Cover the bowl and let the shrimp marinate for 30 to 60 minutes.

3. Cook the shrimp in a medium pan over medium heat until they start to turn pink, 5 to 7 minutes. Flip them over to cook the other side for an additional 5 to 7 minutes. The shrimp will decrease in size as they cook. Make sure that the shrimp reach an internal temperature of 145°F before removing them from the pan.

Tip: Add these shrimp to the Butter Lettuce Salad with Shrimp (page 50) or enjoy them alongside the Three-Grain Ancient Blend on page 107.

* If you can, marinate and thaw the shrimp overnight in the refrigerator.

Lentil and Quinoa "Meat"balls

Prep time: 10 minutes | Cook time: 45 to 50 minutes

Lentils are an excellent choice for vegetarians. They are high in iron, folate, and protein, among other nutrients. The egg, almond meal, and feta cheese keep the "meat"balls intact.

Yield: 3 to 4 servings
Serving size:

3 to 4 meatballs

GLUTEN-FREE, SOY-FREE,
VEGETARIAN, GOOD FOR
POSTPARTUM RECOVERY

⅓ cup uncooked
    quinoa, rinsed
⅔ cup water
½ cup uncooked lentils, rinsed
1½ cups vegetable broth
1 teaspoon avocado oil
½ large red onion, chopped
4 garlic cloves, minced
½ cup almond meal
1 teaspoon Italian seasoning
½ teaspoon salt
½ teaspoon freshly ground
    black pepper
⅓ cup feta cheese
    (pasteurized if currently
    pregnant)
1 large egg, beaten

1. Preheat the oven to 400°F. Line a rimmed baking sheet with parchment paper and set aside.

2. Add the quinoa and water to a small pot and bring to a boil. Reduce the heat to low, cover, and simmer for 20 minutes.

3. Add the lentils and the broth to another small pot and bring to a boil. Reduce the heat to low, cover, and simmer for 20 minutes.

4. Heat the oil in a small sauté pan over medium heat and sauté the onion until it begins to brown, 3 to 5 minutes. Add the garlic and sauté for another 1 to 2 minutes.

5. When the quinoa and lentils are done, transfer them both to a medium mixing bowl.

6. Add the onion and garlic, almond meal, Italian seasoning, salt, pepper, cheese, and egg, stirring to combine.

7. Form the mixture into 1-inch balls and place them on the prepared baking sheet.

8. Roast in the oven for 20 minutes, or until the balls start to turn golden brown.

Per serving: Calories: 439; Total fat: 22g; Saturated fat: 5g; Carbohydrate: 40g; Sugar: 2g; Fiber: 8g; Protein: 22g; Sodium: 988mg; Cholesterol: 71mg

ONE-POT BEEF AND BROCCOLI

Prep time: 20 minutes | Cook time: 20 minutes

Beef and broccoli is one of my favorite dishes when I eat at Asian restaurants, but most of the time it is loaded with salt and sugar. Making it at home is simple and the result is more nutritious.

Yield: 4 to 5 servings
Serving size: 1 cup

DAIRY-FREE, GLUTEN-FREE,
NUT-FREE, ENERGY
ENHANCER, GOOD FOR
LEG CRAMPS, GOOD FOR
POSTPARTUM RECOVERY

1 tablespoon avocado oil
1 pound steak, sliced into
    ¼-inch pieces
4 garlic cloves, minced
½ cup beef broth
4 cups fresh broccoli, chopped
⅓ cup soy sauce
2 tablespoons sesame oil
1 teaspoon ground ginger
4 tablespoons water
2 tablespoons cornstarch or
    arrowroot powder

Per serving: Calories: 401;
Total fat: 23g; Saturated fat: 7g;
Carbohydrate: 12g; Sugar: 2g;
Fiber: 3g; Protein: 36g; Sodium:
1419mg; Cholesterol: 81mg

1. Heat the oil in a large pot over medium heat and cook the steak for about 4 minutes. Add the garlic and cook for an additional minute.

2. Add the broth and broccoli to the pot. Cover with a lid and steam the broccoli for 10 minutes.

3. Meanwhile, in a small bowl, whisk together the soy sauce, sesame oil, ginger, water, and cornstarch.

4. Once the broccoli is tender, add the soy sauce mixture to the pot. Stir everything together and cook until the sauce begins to thicken.

5. Serve as is or over brown rice or riced cauliflower (a great alternative if you have gestational diabetes).

Tip: Follow the same steps to make this dish in an Instant Pot®. Use the sauté function to cook the meat and then switch to the steam function after adding the broccoli. Steam for 7 minutes, quick release the steam, select sauté again, and add the soy sauce mixture. Stir until the sauce thickens.

Rainbow Chard–Stuffed Chicken Breasts

Prep time: 15 minutes | Cook time: 35 to 50 minutes

A lot of people limit their consumption of leafy greens to spinach, kale, and romaine lettuce, but there are many others to try. Rainbow chard, which is showcased in this recipe, is one example. It is colorful, nutrient-dense, and delicious.

Yield: 3 servings

Serving size:
1 chicken breast

GLUTEN-FREE, NUT-FREE, GESTATIONAL DIABETES– FRIENDLY, GOOD FOR PRE-CONCEPTION, GOOD FOR SWELLING

1 tablespoon butter or
　1 teaspoon avocado oil
1 bunch rainbow
　chard, chopped
3 boneless chicken breasts
4 ounces Parmesan
　cheese, grated
Salt, for seasoning
Freshly ground black pepper,
　for seasoning

1. Preheat the oven to 400°F.

2. Heat the butter in a medium sauté pan over medium heat and sauté the chard for 5 to 7 minutes.

3. While the chard is cooking, cut 2- to 3-inch pockets into the center of each of the chicken breasts. This is where you will put the stuffing.

4. Once the chard is sautéed, combine it with the Parmesan cheese in a large bowl, stirring until the cheese is melted.

5. Stuff the chicken breasts with the chard mixture and season them on both sides with salt and pepper.

6. Place the chicken breasts in a 9-by-9-inch baking dish or on a baking sheet. Bake in the oven for 30 to 40 minutes.

Per serving: Calories: 212; Total fat: 9g; Saturated fat: 4g; Carbohydrate: 5g; Sugar: 1g; Fiber: 1g; Protein: 30g; Sodium: 799mg; Cholesterol: 89mg

SLOW-COOKED PULLED PORK

Prep time: 5 minutes | Cook time: 8 hours

This is a slow cooker recipe, so do the prep work before you go to work in the morning. Delicious smells will greet you when you arrive home. This dish is perfect for large families or for a small social gathering.

Yield: 8 servings

Serving size: 3 to 4 ounces

DAIRY-FREE, GLUTEN-FREE, NUT-FREE, SOY-FREE, GOOD FOR POSTPARTUM RECOVERY, KID-FRIENDLY

1 medium yellow onion, sliced
4 garlic cloves, minced
1 orange, juiced
2 tablespoons paprika
2 teaspoons Italian seasoning
1 teaspoon salt
1 teaspoon freshly ground black pepper
½ teaspoon cumin
1 teaspoon ground mustard
4½ pounds bone-in pork shoulder roast

Per serving: Calories: 610; Total fat: 47g; Saturated fat: 16g; Carbohydrate: 6g; Sugar: 3g; Fiber: 2g; Protein: 39g; Sodium: 443mg; Cholesterol: 116mg

1. Add all the ingredients to the slow cooker.

2. Place the lid on the slow cooker, set the heat to low, and cook for 8 hours.

3. Remove the meat from the pot and place it on a large plate. Use a fork to shred the meat.

4. To add extra moisture and flavor, top the meat with the remaining juice from the slow cooker.

Tip: Pair this recipe with Simple Coleslaw (page 106).

Half Noodle Lasagna

Prep time: 15 minutes | Cook time: 35 minutes

I normally use spinach in pasta dishes, but for this one, I went with zucchini. If you have gestational diabetes, try eliminating or reducing noodles to decrease the carb content.

Yield: 8 servings

Serving size:

1 (2-inch) square

DAIRY-FREE, NUT-FREE, SOY-FREE, GOOD FOR POSTPARTUM RECOVERY, KID-FRIENDLY

1 teaspoon avocado oil

½ large yellow onion, diced

1 pound ground beef

2 teaspoons Italian seasoning

2 cups marinara or tomato sauce

8 large lasagna noodles

1 cup ricotta cheese

1½ cups mozzarella cheese, divided

2 large zucchinis, sliced into thin strips lengthwise

Per serving: Calories: 391; Total fat: 13g; Saturated fat: 6g; Carbohydrate: 42g; Sugar: 5g; Fiber: 2g; Protein: 28g; Sodium: 544mg; Cholesterol: 82mg

1. Preheat the oven to 375°F.

2. Heat the oil in a medium sauté pan over medium heat and sauté the onion for about 3 minutes.

3. Add the ground beef and Italian seasoning to the pan and cook until the meat is no longer pink. Once the meat is cooked through, add the marinara to the pan, stirring well to combine.

4. Fill a medium pot with water and bring to a boil over high heat. Add the lasagna noodles and cook according to the package directions.

5. In a medium mixing bowl, combine the ricotta with 1 cup of the mozzarella.

6. In a 9-by-13-inch baking pan, add half of the meat mixture in one thin layer. Cover with half of the cheese mixture. Then layer half of the zucchini slices, 4 lasagna noodles, the other half of the meat mixture, more cheese, the rest of the zucchini, and the remaining four noodles.

7. Bake in the oven for 15 minutes. Add the remaining ½ cup of mozzarella and cook for another 5 to 7 minutes or until the cheese on top is melted and starting to brown.

Tip: This is a nice freezer-friendly meal. Pre-cut the squares and freeze them individually or together for after the baby comes. It will last up to 4 months in the freezer. Thaw overnight in the refrigerator before reheating.

Baked Chicken Legs

Prep time: 5 minutes | Cook time: 30 to 40 minutes

This is one of my go-to protein options for a weeknight dinner. These baked chicken legs are simple and go with nearly every side dish in this book!

Yield: 5 servings

Serving size: 1 to 2 chicken legs

DAIRY-FREE, GLUTEN-FREE, NUT-FREE, SOY-FREE, GESTATIONAL DIABETES–FRIENDLY, GOOD FOR PRE-CONCEPTION, KID-FRIENDLY

5 to 6 chicken legs

½ teaspoon salt

½ teaspoon freshly ground black pepper

½ teaspoon garlic powder

1. Preheat the oven to 400°F.

2. Place the chicken legs (no need to remove the skin) in a 9-by-9-inch baking dish.

3. In a small bowl, combine the salt, pepper, and garlic powder and sprinkle half the seasoning on one side of the legs. Flip the legs over and use the rest of the seasoning to evenly coat them.

4. Bake in the oven for 30 to 40 minutes, or until a kitchen thermometer shows they have reached an internal temperature of 165°F.

Per serving: Calories: 295; Total fat: 20g; Saturated fat: 6g; Carbohydrate: 0g; Sugar: 0g; Fiber: 0g; Protein: 30g; Sodium: 359mg; Cholesterol: 133mg

Cumin Chicken and Black Beans

Prep time: 5 minutes | Cook time: 45 minutes to 1 hour

If you are in the mood for Mexican but aren't interested in eating out, this is your dish. It's basic but really tasty.

Yield: 6 servings

Serving size: 1 chicken thigh with ½ cup black beans

GLUTEN-FREE, NUT-FREE, SOY-FREE, GESTATIONAL DIABETES–FRIENDLY, GOOD FOR PRE-CONCEPTION, KID-FRIENDLY

6 chicken thighs

½ teaspoon salt

½ teaspoon freshly ground black pepper

½ teaspoon cumin

1 (15-ounce) can refried black beans

8 ounces salsa

⅓ cup Mexican blend cheese (optional)

Per serving: Calories: 328; Total fat: 21g; Saturated fat: 6g; Carbohydrate: 9g; Sugar: 1g; Fiber: 3g; Protein: 26g; Sodium: 580mg; Cholesterol: 111mg

1. Preheat the oven to 375°F.

2. Place the chicken thighs (no need to remove the skin) in a 9-by-13-inch baking pan.

3. In a small bowl, combine the salt, pepper, and cumin. Coat the chicken evenly using all the seasoning.

4. Add the black beans and salsa to the pan, around and on top of the chicken in a random fashion.

5. Bake in the oven for 45 minutes to an hour, or until a kitchen thermometer shows the internal temperature of the chicken has reached 165°F. If you are adding the cheese, sprinkle it on top of the chicken when it has baked for 35 minutes.

Tip: Make this dish dairy-free by omitting the cheese topping.

Almond-Crusted Cod

Prep time: 5 minutes, plus overnight to marinate | Cook time: 20 minutes

I used to dislike fish until I started trying new ways to cook it. A little crunch on the outside makes fish taste that much better.

Yield: 3 to 4 servings
Serving size:
1 (3- to 4-ounce) cod fillet

DAIRY-FREE, GLUTEN-FREE, SOY-FREE, GESTATIONAL DIABETES–FRIENDLY, GOOD FOR LACTATION, KID-FRIENDLY

1 pound cod fillets, fresh or frozen
Juice of ½ lemon
1 large egg, beaten
½ teaspoon salt
½ teaspoon freshly ground black pepper
¾ cup almond meal
Slivered almonds (optional)

1. Marinate the fish in the lemon juice overnight in a baking dish. (This will add more flavor to the fish.)

2. When you are ready to cook the fish, preheat the oven to 375°F and line a baking sheet with parchment paper.

3. In a small bowl, combine the egg, salt, and pepper.

4. In a medium bowl, add the almond meal.

5. Dip each fillet in the egg mixture and then coat with the almond meal. Place the coated fillets on the prepared baking sheet.

6. Bake the cod in the oven for 20 minutes or until a kitchen thermometer shows the internal temperature has reached 145°F.

7. Sprinkle slivered almonds on top of the fish before serving, if desired.

Per serving: Calories: 312; Total fat: 16g; Saturated fat: 2g; Carbohydrate: 6g; Sugar: 0g; Fiber: 3g; Protein: 34g; Sodium: 525mg; Cholesterol: 108mg

ROASTED VEGGIE WRAP

Prep time: 20 minutes | Cook time: 15 minutes

Calling all veggie lovers! This wrap comes together quickly, and any left-over green spread can be used on sandwiches, as a salad dressing, or to baste meats.

Yield: 4 servings

Serving size: 1 wrap

DAIRY-FREE, GLUTEN-FREE, NUT-FREE, SOY-FREE, VEGAN, GOOD FOR CONSTIPATION, QUICK

FOR THE SPREAD

1 medium avocado
¼ cup fresh basil
¼ cup fresh parsley
2 garlic cloves
2 tablespoons scallions
2 tablespoons extra-virgin olive oil
Juice of ½ lemon
½ teaspoon salt

FOR THE WRAP

1 tablespoon avocado oil
1 red bell pepper, seeded and sliced
½ medium red onion, sliced
1 cup sliced Portobello mushrooms
1 (14-ounce) can artichoke hearts, drained
2 spinach wraps
2 cups mixed greens
½ cup Roasted Chickpeas (page 114; optional)

TO MAKE THE SPREAD

In a food processor, blend all the ingredients for the spread until smooth.

TO MAKE THE WRAPS

1. Heat the oil in a medium skillet over medium heat and cook the bell pepper and onion for about 8 minutes.

2. Add the mushrooms to the skillet and sauté with the other veggies for about 3 minutes.

3. Add the artichokes to the skillet with the other veggies. Sauté for another 2 to 3 minutes. Remove from the heat.

4. Lay the wraps on individual plates and add 1 tablespoon of the spread to each wrap.

5. Divide the greens and all the veggies from the skillet evenly between the wraps.

6. Sprinkle 2 tablespoons of roasted chickpeas on each wrap, if desired.

Per serving: Calories: 333; Total fat: 22g; Saturated fat: 3g; Carbohydrate: 30g; Sugar: 3g; Fiber: 6g; Protein: 7g; Sodium: 691mg; Cholesterol: 0mg

CREATE YOUR OWN FLATBREAD

Prep time: 10 minutes | Cook time: 15 minutes

My husband and I can never agree on pizza toppings. For this reason, individual "create your own" pizzas are amazing. This recipe is fun to make on a weekend night with your kids, too.

Yield: 1 flatbread pizza

Serving size:

1 flatbread pizza

NUT-FREE, SOY-FREE, GOOD FOR PRECONCEPTION, KID-FRIENDLY, QUICK

FOR THE BASE

Tortilla, wrap, English muffin, or naan

FOR THE SAUCE

½ cup marinara sauce, ½ cup pesto sauce (see page 49), and ½ cup green spread (see page 82), **OR** 2 tablespoons extra-virgin olive oil

FOR THE TOPPINGS

3 artichoke hearts, ¼ cup sautéed red onion, and 2 prosciutto slices; **OR**

3 ounces diced chicken with pesto sauce; **OR**

1 cup sautéed fresh spinach, ½ cup roasted tomatoes, and 1 tablespoon roasted garlic pieces

FOR THE CHEESE

½ cup mozzarella, ¼ cup mozzarella, and ¼ cup Parmesan, **OR** ½ cup ricotta cheese

1. Preheat the oven to 350°F.

2. In a medium skillet over medium heat, sauté any veggie toppings, adding any leafy greens last.

3. Spread your sauce evenly over your base/crust. Add your preferred veggies and then top with your cheese choice.

4. Bake in the oven for approximately 15 minutes.

Per serving: Calories: 342; Total fat: 14g; Saturated fat: 8g; Carbohydrate: 35g; Sugar: 8g; Fiber: 4g; Protein: 20g; Sodium: 675mg; Cholesterol: 45mg

Two-Pan Turkey Dinner

....

Prep time: 5 minutes | Cook time: 20 minutes

Anytime my husband cooks dinner (which isn't often), he makes this meal. This turkey dinner is super simple, and it makes really great lunches for the week.

....

Yield: 6 servings

Serving size: 1 cup turkey and veggies

DAIRY-FREE, GLUTEN-FREE, NUT-FREE, SOY-FREE, ENERGY ENHANCER, GESTATIONAL DIABETES–FRIENDLY, GOOD FOR PRE-CONCEPTION, QUICK

1 teaspoon salt
1 teaspoon freshly ground black pepper
2 tablespoons Italian seasoning
2 tablespoons avocado oil, divided
1 pound ground turkey
1 cup baby carrots, halved
2 cups chopped fresh broccoli
1 bell pepper, any color, seeded and diced
Sriracha sauce (optional)

1. In a small bowl, combine the salt, pepper, and Italian seasoning.

2. Heat 1 tablespoon of oil in a large skillet over medium heat. Add the ground turkey with half of the seasoning mixture.

3. In another large skillet, warm the remaining 1 tablespoon of oil and add the carrots, broccoli, and bell pepper with the other half of the seasoning mixture.

4. Cook the turkey for approximately 20 minutes until it is no longer pink, or a kitchen thermometer shows it has reached 165°F. Cook the veggies until the carrots are tender, about 20 minutes.

5. Serve everything together in one bowl. If you'd like, drizzle on a little Sriracha sauce for extra flavor and spice.

Per serving: Calories: 153; Total fat: 8g; Saturated fat: 2g; Carbohydrate: 5g; Sugar: 2g; Fiber: 2g; Protein: 14g; Sodium: 477mg; Cholesterol: 63mg

Cashew Chicken (or Tempeh) Lettuce Wraps

Prep time: 25 minutes | Cook time: 35 minutes

I love many kinds of lettuce wraps, but these are probably my favorite. They seem complicated when you order them at PF Chang's, but I've simplified them. Don't worry—they are still delicious!

Yield: 4 servings

Serving size: 2 to 3 lettuce wraps

DAIRY-FREE, GLUTEN-FREE, GESTATIONAL DIABETES–FRIENDLY, KID-FRIENDLY

1 tablespoon avocado oil

½ medium yellow onion, diced

½ cup carrots, diced

1 red bell pepper, seeded and diced

3 garlic cloves, minced

1 pound ground chicken

2 tablespoons soy sauce

1 tablespoon rice vinegar

¼ teaspoon ground ginger

¼ teaspoon freshly ground black pepper

1 teaspoon sesame oil

2 teaspoons maple syrup or honey

⅓ cup cashews, chopped

1 head green leaf lettuce or butter lettuce

Per serving: Calories: 318; Total fat: 19g; Saturated fat: 4g; Carbohydrate: 15g; Sugar: 6g; Fiber: 2g; Protein: 23g; Sodium: 536mg; Cholesterol: 96mg

1. Heat the oil in a large skillet over medium heat and sauté the onion. After 3 to 5 minutes, add the carrots and bell pepper and sauté for 5 to 7 minutes. Add the garlic and sauté for an additional 2 to 3 minutes.

2. Add the chicken and cook for approximately 20 minutes until it is no longer pink in the center, or until a kitchen thermometer shows it has reached an internal temperature of 165°F.

3. Meanwhile, in a medium bowl, whisk together the soy sauce, vinegar, ginger, black pepper, sesame oil, and maple syrup.

4. Once the chicken is cooked, remove it from the skillet and transfer it to a medium bowl. Add the cashews and the sauce and mix together.

5. Scoop about ¼ cup of the filling into one leaf of lettuce. Roll up and enjoy!

Tip: To make this recipe vegan, use an 8-ounce block of tempeh instead of chicken. Cut the tempeh into ½-inch cubes and place them in a food processor. Pulse until the consistency resembles ground chicken. All the other steps in the process remain the same.

Mahi-Mahi Fish Tacos

Prep time: 15 minutes, plus 20 minutes to marinate | Cook time: 15 minutes

You'll want to invite your friends over for taco Tuesday to try this dish. Mahi-mahi has 20 grams of protein per 3 ounces and is an excellent source of selenium and B vitamins.

Yield: 1 serving
Serving size: 2 tacos

GLUTEN-FREE, NUT-FREE, SOY-FREE, GESTATIONAL DIABETES–FRIENDLY

Juice of 1 lime

1 tablespoon minced garlic

2 teaspoons taco seasoning or chili powder

8 ounces mahi-mahi

1 tablespoon avocado oil

2 corn tortillas

1 tablespoon chopped fresh cilantro

1 cup shredded green cabbage

¼ cup diced scallions

1 medium avocado, peeled, pitted, and sliced

Sour cream and Cheddar cheese, for topping (optional)

1. In a small bowl, whisk together the lime juice, garlic, and taco seasoning.

2. Add the mahi-mahi to a shallow pan and coat each fillet with the seasoning blend. Marinate the fish in the refrigerator for 20 minutes.

3. Heat the oil in a cast-iron skillet over medium heat and cook the fillets for approximately 15 minutes, flipping occasionally, until the fish flakes easily, or until it has reached an internal temperature of 145°F.

4. Once the fish is done cooking, transfer the fillets to a plate and use a fork to shred them into bite-size pieces.

5. Divide the fish between the corn tortillas. Top with the cilantro, cabbage, scallions, and avocado. Add sour cream and Cheddar cheese, if desired.

Per serving: Calories: 295; Total fat: 15g; Saturated fat: 2g; Carbohydrate: 27g; Sugar: 3g; Fiber: 8g; Protein: 18g; Sodium: 95mg; Cholesterol: 27mg

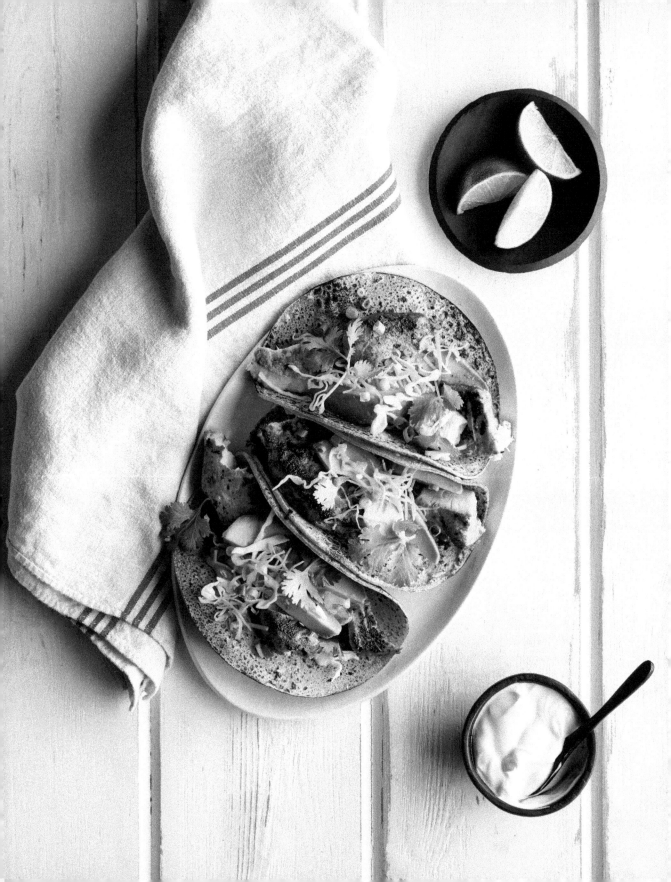

Lamb Kabobs

Prep time: 15 minutes, plus 30 minutes to 3 hours to marinate
Cook time: 12 to 20 minutes

Lamb is something I cook to add variety to my proteins. Lamb is rich in B vitamins (especially B$_{12}$), zinc, choline, and glycine.

Yield: 6 servings
Serving size: 1 skewer

DAIRY-FREE, GLUTEN-FREE, NUT-FREE, SOY-FREE, GESTATIONAL DIABETES–FRIENDLY, KID-FRIENDLY

FOR THE MARINADE

¼ cup olive oil
2 tablespoons lemon juice
2 garlic cloves, minced
1 teaspoon paprika
1 teaspoon ground cumin
1 teaspoon salt, plus extra for seasoning
½ teaspoon oregano
¼ teaspoon freshly ground black pepper, plus extra for seasoning

FOR THE KABOBS

2 pounds boneless leg of a lamb, cut into 1- to 2-inch pieces
1 medium red onion, chopped into large pieces
3 bell peppers, in assorted colors, seeded and chopped into large pieces
8 ounces whole white button mushrooms

TO MAKE THE MARINADE

1. Combine the marinade ingredients in a medium bowl.

2. Add the lamb and marinate in the refrigerator for 30 minutes to 3 hours.

3. If you are using wooden skewers to make the kabobs, soak them in water for 30 minutes while the lamb is marinating.

TO MAKE THE KABOBS

1. Slide the pieces of lamb, onion, and bell pepper and whole mushrooms onto 8 metal or wooden skewers, alternating each food as you go. There should be about four pieces of lamb on each skewer.

2. Sprinkle the skewers with a little extra salt and pepper or drizzle the leftover marinade on top.

3. You can either cook the skewers on a grill or bake them in the oven. To bake, preheat the oven to 375°F, place the kabobs on a baking sheet, and bake for 15 to 20 minutes. To grill, place the skewers on a metal grate and cook for 12 to 15 minutes, rotating halfway through.

Per serving: Calories: 460; Total fat: 34g; Saturated fat: 12g; Carbohydrate: 9g; Sugar: 4g; Fiber: 2g; Protein: 29g; Sodium: 485mg; Cholesterol: 107mg

Spinach Parmesan Spaghetti Squash

Prep time: 10 minutes | Cook time: 50 minutes

Cooking spaghetti squash is much easier than you might think. Be aware that if you are craving real pasta, this squash will likely not satisfy your craving. It does make what looks like thin noodles, but the texture is not pasta-like. Don't worry though—this dish is still very yummy!

Yield: 2 to 3 servings

Serving size: 1 cup

GLUTEN-FREE, NUT-FREE, SOY-FREE, VEGETARIAN, GESTATIONAL DIABETES–FRIENDLY, GOOD FOR LEG CRAMPS, GOOD FOR POSTPARTUM RECOVERY

1 spaghetti squash, cut in half lengthwise

2 teaspoons extra-virgin olive oil, divided

Salt, for seasoning

Freshly ground black pepper, for seasoning

1 teaspoon fresh thyme

3 garlic cloves, minced

5 ounces fresh spinach

½ cup heavy cream

1 tablespoon cream cheese

½ cup grated Parmesan cheese

Per serving: Calories: 455; Total fat: 36g; Saturated fat: 20g; Carbohydrate: 25g; Sugar: 0g; Fiber: 2g; Protein: 15g; Sodium: 475mg; Cholesterol: 107mg

1. Preheat the oven to 400°F.

2. Place the squash halves on a baking sheet and rub the bottom of each half with ½ teaspoon of the oil. Sprinkle the insides of the squash with salt, pepper, and thyme. Roast the squash, cut-side up, for about 40 minutes.

3. Meanwhile, heat the remaining 1 teaspoon of oil in a skillet over medium heat. Sauté the garlic for 1 to 2 minutes.

4. Add the spinach, heavy cream, cream cheese, and Parmesan cheese to the skillet.

5. Once the spinach begins to wilt, remove the skillet from the heat.

6. Remove the squash from the oven and let it cool for a few minutes.

7. Use a fork to scrape the inside of each squash. As the squash separates from the skin, it'll look like angel-hair pasta noodles.

8. Top the squash "noodles" with the spinach and cheese mixture.

Tip: Add Lemony Garlic Shrimp (page 73) to enhance this recipe. You can also incorporate artichoke hearts by adding them to the skillet with the spinach in step 4.

Pan-Seared Rainbow Trout

Prep time: 10 minutes | Cook time: 15 minutes

It is challenging to get all of your vitamin D through food and sun exposure. Fish—especially rainbow trout—is one of the only dietary sources of vitamin D. It is also a good source of vitamin B12 and DHA.

Yield: 4 servings
Serving size: 3 ounces

GLUTEN-FREE, NUT-FREE, SOY-FREE, ENERGY ENHANCER, GESTATIONAL DIABETES–FRIENDLY, GOOD FOR LACTATION, QUICK

1½ pounds skinless trout
¼ teaspoon salt
¼ teaspoon freshly ground black pepper
1 tablespoon Italian seasoning
1 tablespoon extra-virgin olive oil
2 tablespoons minced garlic
2 tablespoons butter
Juice of ½ lemon
2 tablespoons chopped fresh parsley

Per serving: Calories: 339; Total fat: 19g; Saturated fat: 4g; Carbohydrate: 2g; Sugar: 0g; Fiber: 1g; Protein: 37g; Sodium: 193mg; Cholesterol: 18mg

1. Season the fish with the salt, pepper, and Italian seasoning.

2. Heat the oil in a large skillet over medium heat and cook the fish for 3 to 5 minutes.

3. Flip the fish and cook for an additional 3 to 5 minutes until the fish flakes easily, or until the fish has reached an internal temperature of 145°F.

4. Remove the fish from the skillet and set aside.

5. In the same skillet, add the garlic, butter, and lemon juice. Cook for 1 to 2 minutes then turn off the heat and add the chopped parsley.

6. Add the fish back to the skillet and spoon the sauce over the top of the fish before serving.

Tip: Add Cauliflower Mash (page 108) or Roasted Broccoli with Shallots (page 102) to make a complete nutrient-dense dinner.

Easy Black Bean Burger

Prep time: 20 minutes | Cook time: 10 to 15 minutes

Store-bought frozen veggie burgers usually contain unnecessary ingredients and fillers. Making black bean burgers at home isn't challenging and allows for creativity. You can try using different beans or add other veggies.

Yield: 4 servings
Serving size: 1 patty

DAIRY-FREE, GLUTEN-FREE, NUT-FREE, SOY-FREE, VEGAN, GOOD FOR CONSTIPATION, GOOD FOR LACTATION, QUICK

1 teaspoon extra-virgin olive oil, divided
1 shallot, chopped
1 small zucchini, grated
1 (15.5-ounce) can black beans, drained and rinsed
¼ cup gluten-free rolled oats
2 tablespoons ground flaxseed
1 teaspoon dried oregano
1 teaspoon dried basil
¼ teaspoon salt
¼ cup fresh parsley
Optional toppings and extras: burger bun or toast, avocado toppings, green spread (see page 82), tomato slices, and Cotija cheese

Per serving: Calories: 112; Total fat: 3g; Saturated fat: 0g; Carbohydrate: 16g; Sugar: 1g; Fiber: 6g; Protein: 5g; Sodium: 263mg; Cholesterol: 0mg

1. Heat ½ teaspoon of oil in a skillet over medium heat and sauté the shallot for 2 to 3 minutes.

2. Roll the grated zucchini in paper towels and squeeze out excess moisture over the sink.

3. Add the sautéed shallot, beans, zucchini, oats, flaxseed, oregano, basil, salt, and parsley to a food processor and blend until smooth. Shape into 4 round, 2-inch patties.

4. Place the same skillet that you used to sauté the shallot over medium heat. Add the remaining oil and the patties. Cook for 3 to 5 minutes on each side.

5. Add the toppings of your choice.

Tip: Make a double batch and freeze these patties for up to four months. Thaw them in the refrigerator before frying.

Mediterranean Roasted Salmon

Prep time: 15 minutes | Cook time: 10 to 15 minutes

Before, during, and after pregnancy, you'll want to include salmon in your diet. This recipe delivers critical nutrients and can be cooked in one skillet.

Yield: 2 servings

Serving size:
1 salmon fillet

DAIRY-FREE, GLUTEN-FREE, NUT-FREE, SOY-FREE, GESTATIONAL DIABETES– FRIENDLY, MAY HELP WITH HEADACHES

½ teaspoon dried basil
½ teaspoon garlic powder
½ teaspoon dried rosemary
½ teaspoon salt
¼ teaspoon freshly ground black pepper
2 (4-ounce) salmon fillets
2 tablespoons extra-virgin olive oil, divided
1 medium fennel bulb, chopped
1 cup chopped cherry tomatoes

1. In a small bowl, combine the basil, garlic powder, rosemary, salt, and pepper.

2. Sprinkle the seasoning mixture on both salmon fillets.

3. Heat 1 tablespoon oil in a large skillet over medium heat and cook the salmon, skin-side up, for 4 to 5 minutes.

4. Add the remaining 1 tablespoon of olive oil to the skillet. Flip the salmon and then add the fennel and tomatoes to the skillet.

5. Cook for an additional 6 to 8 minutes. You'll know the fish is done when it flakes easily, or a kitchen thermometer shows the fish has reached an internal temperature of 145°F.

Per serving: Calories: 336; Total fat: 19g; Saturated fat: 3g; Carbohydrate: 13g; Sugar: 3g; Fiber: 5g; Protein: 29g; Sodium: 171mg; Cholesterol: 60mg

Turkey Arugula Pasta

Prep time: 15 minutes | Cook time: 35 minutes

Sun-dried tomatoes add a wonderful flavor dimension to this pasta dish. My mom loved this recipe so much the first time she tried it that she made it two weeks in a row.

Yield: 4 to 6 servings
Serving size: 1 cup

DAIRY-FREE, NUT-FREE, SOY-FREE, GOOD FOR POSTPARTUM RECOVERY, KID-FRIENDLY

8 ounces rotini pasta
¼ teaspoon dried basil
¼ teaspoon dried rosemary
¼ teaspoon garlic powder
½ teaspoon salt
⅛ teaspoon freshly ground black pepper
2 tablespoons extra-virgin olive oil
1 shallot, chopped
1 pound ground turkey
10 plain sun-dried tomatoes, chopped
1 teaspoon minced garlic
2 tablespoons balsamic vinegar
2 cups arugula

Per serving: Calories: 492; Total fat: 18g; Saturated fat: 4g; Carbohydrate: 55g; Sugar: 10g; Fiber: 6g; Protein: 30g; Sodium: 359mg; Cholesterol: 90mg

1. Cook the pasta according to the package directions.

2. In a small bowl, combine the basil, rosemary, garlic powder, salt, and pepper.

3. Heat the oil in a large skillet over medium heat and sauté the shallot for 2 to 3 minutes.

4. Add the turkey and the seasoning blend to the skillet. Cook the turkey for approximately 20 minutes until it is no longer pink, or until a kitchen thermometer shows it has reached an internal temperature of 165°F.

5. In the bowl you used to make the seasoning blend, combine the sun-dried tomatoes, minced garlic, and balsamic vinegar.

6. Add the cooked pasta and cooked meat to a large bowl and combine with the sun-dried tomato mixture.

7. Add the arugula and toss everything together before serving.

Tip: Try the Traditional Caprese Salad (page 117) as an appetizer for this dish.

Tofu Stir-Fry

Prep time: 20 minutes | Cook time: 30 minutes

If you're not a vegetarian, tofu probably isn't your thing. But even if you prefer meat, it's worth trying. Make sure you buy tofu that has been fortified with calcium for additional nutrients.

Yield: 4 servings
Serving size: 1½ cups stir-fry

DAIRY-FREE, NUT-FREE, VEGETARIAN, GOOD FOR CONSTIPATION

½ cup uncooked brown rice
1 cup water
7 ounces extra firm tofu
2 tablespoons soy sauce
½ teaspoon ground ginger
2 teaspoons sesame oil
1 tablespoon avocado oil
3 cups fresh or frozen stir-fry veggies
2 large eggs
1 tablespoon sesame seeds

1. In a medium pot or rice cooker, add the rice and water and bring to a boil. Reduce the heat to low, cover, and cook for 30 minutes.

2. Drain the water from the tofu and pat it dry with paper towels. Cut the tofu into 1- to 2-inch cubes.

3. In a medium bowl, add the tofu, soy sauce, ginger, and sesame oil. Let the mixture sit for 7 to 10 minutes.

4. Heat the oil in a large skillet over medium heat and sauté the veggies for approximately 10 minutes.

5. After the tofu has set with the sauce, add it to the skillet with the veggies and cook for 10 to 15 minutes, until the tofu is golden brown and crispy around the edges. Don't flip or mix the tofu too much or it will fall apart.

6. In the same bowl you used for the tofu, whisk the 2 eggs. Microwave them for 1 to 2 minutes. Use a fork or knife to chop the egg into small pieces, and add them to the skillet.

7. To serve, fill each bowl with ½ cup brown rice, 1 cup veggies, and 5 to 6 pieces of tofu. Top with sesame seeds.

Per serving: Calories: 268; Total fat: 12g; Saturated fat: 2g; Carbohydrate: 25g; Sugar: 3g; Fiber: 3g; Protein: 13g; Sodium: 517mg; Cholesterol: 82mg

SAUSAGE WITH APPLE SAUERKRAUT AND POTATOES

Prep time: 10 minutes | Cook time: 30 to 45 minutes

Sauerkraut is a great addition to your prenatal diet because it is fermented, which means it contains probiotics. A healthy intake of probiotics during pregnancy has been linked to a number of benefits, including improved digestion and increased immunity from certain infections.

Yield: 4 servings
Serving size: 1 cup

GLUTEN-FREE, NUT-FREE, SOY-FREE, GOOD FOR POSTPARTUM RECOVERY

6 medium red potatoes, chopped into 1-inch cubes
3 tablespoons butter
1 medium sweet onion, sliced
2 medium apples, cut into ⅛- to ¼-inch slices
1 tablespoon lemon juice
8 ounces sauerkraut
½ cup unsweetened apple juice
1 teaspoon caraway seeds
½ teaspoon crushed fennel seed
1 pound sausage links
Salt, for seasoning
Freshly ground black pepper, for seasoning

1. Place the potatoes in a medium glass bowl and microwave them for 8 minutes.

2. Heat the butter in a large skillet over medium heat and sauté the onion for 5 minutes. Add the potatoes and cook for an additional 8 to 10 minutes.

3. In a large bowl, toss the apples with the lemon juice. Add the apples, sauerkraut, apple juice, caraway seeds, and fennel seed to the skillet with the onion and bring to a boil. Reduce the heat, cover, and simmer for 15 minutes.

4. Cook the sausage links in the microwave for 5 to 7 minutes, rotating every 30 seconds, or sauté them in the skillet for 10 to 15 minutes until fully cooked. Cut the sausage into slices, serve with the sauerkraut and potatoes, and season with salt and pepper.

Per serving: Calories: 567; Total fat: 19g; Saturated fat: 9g; Carbohydrate: 78g; Sugar: 21g; Fiber: 11g; Protein: 26g; Sodium: 1105mg; Cholesterol: 57mg

BEEF STEW

Prep time: 15 minutes | Cook time: 2 hours

This is probably my family's favorite fall and winter meal. I like to try new vegetables in it.

Yield: 6 to 8 servings

Serving size: 1½ cups

DAIRY-FREE, NUT-FREE, SOY-FREE, ENERGY ENHANCER, GOOD FOR POSTPARTUM RECOVERY, KID-FRIENDLY

1 tablespoon extra-virgin olive oil

2 shallots, chopped

1 to 1½ pounds stew meat

4 cups (32 ounces) broth (veggie, beef, or chicken)

1 tablespoon tomato paste

½ teaspoon salt

¼ teaspoon freshly ground black pepper

1 teaspoon paprika

1 bay leaf

1 (16-ounce) bag baby carrots

1 pound tiny white potatoes

1 cup peas, fresh or frozen

2 tablespoons flour

Per serving: Calories: 316; Total fat: 13g; Saturated fat: 5g; Carbohydrate: 25g; Sugar: 6g; Fiber: 5g; Protein: 23g; Sodium: 816mg; Cholesterol: 53mg

1. Heat the oil in a large stock pot over medium-high heat and sauté the shallots for 3 to 4 minutes.

2. Add the stew meat to the pot and cook until just browned, about 10 minutes.

3. Add the broth, tomato paste, salt, pepper, paprika, and bay leaf and bring to a boil. Cover, lower the heat to low, and cook for an hour.

4. After an hour, add the carrots and potatoes to the pot. Cover and cook for another 30 to 45 minutes, until the carrots and potatoes are tender.

5. Add the peas to the pot.

6. Ladle out a quarter of the liquid from the pot and transfer it to a separate bowl. Add the flour and stir to combine.

7. Pour the gravy mixture back into the pot and stir until the stew thickens.

Tip: You can make this recipe in 30 minutes in an Instant Pot®! Use the sauté function to sauté the shallots and cook the stew meat. Once the meat is cooked, add all the other ingredients except the flour. Select the stew function and normal pressure, seal the lid, and set the timer for 25 minutes. Once the stew is done, quick release the steam and then open the lid. Select the sauté function again and complete steps 6 and 7.

Savory Meatballs with Egg Noodles

Prep time: 35 minutes | Cook time: 20 to 30 minutes

Plain buttered noodles may help get you through bouts of nausea during the first trimester, but when your nausea subsides, try adding some flair to your noodles with this recipe!

Yield: 6 servings
Serving size: 1 cup pasta, 3 meatballs

NUT-FREE, SOY-FREE, GOOD FOR POSTPARTUM RECOVERY, KID-FRIENDLY

12 ounces egg noodles
1 pound ground beef
½ cup chopped onion
1 tablespoon minced garlic
1 teaspoon dried oregano
½ teaspoon salt
¼ teaspoon freshly ground black pepper
1 large egg
1 tablespoon extra-virgin olive oil
5 tablespoons butter
3 tablespoons flour
2 cups beef broth
1½ cups heavy cream
½ tablespoon Worcestershire sauce
1 teaspoon Dijon mustard
¼ cup chopped fresh parsley, for garnish (optional)

Per serving: Calories: 682; Total fat: 43g; Saturated fat: 23g; Carbohydrate: 48g; Sugar: 2g; Fiber: 2g; Protein: 27g; Sodium: 642mg; Cholesterol: 229mg

1. Cook the noodles according to the package directions.

2. In a large bowl combine the beef, onion, garlic, oregano, salt, pepper, and egg. Form the mixture into 1-inch balls.

3. Heat the oil in a large skillet over medium heat and cook the meatballs for 20 to 30 minutes until they are no longer pink in the center, or a kitchen thermometer shows the internal temperature has reached 165°F. Transfer the meatballs from the skillet to a plate.

4. Heat the butter in the same large skillet over medium-low heat and add the flour, stirring constantly for about 2 minutes.

5. Slowly add the beef broth. Then add the heavy cream, Worcestershire sauce, and Dijon mustard. Bring the mixture to a simmer.

6. Add the meatballs back to the skillet and cook for an additional 3 to 5 minutes.

7. Top the cooked noodles with the saucy meatballs and garnish with fresh parsley, if desired.

Tip: Bread crumbs aren't absolutely necessary for making meatballs hold together—this is what the egg is for in this recipe. If you are having trouble getting your meatballs to hold together, try adding almond meal.

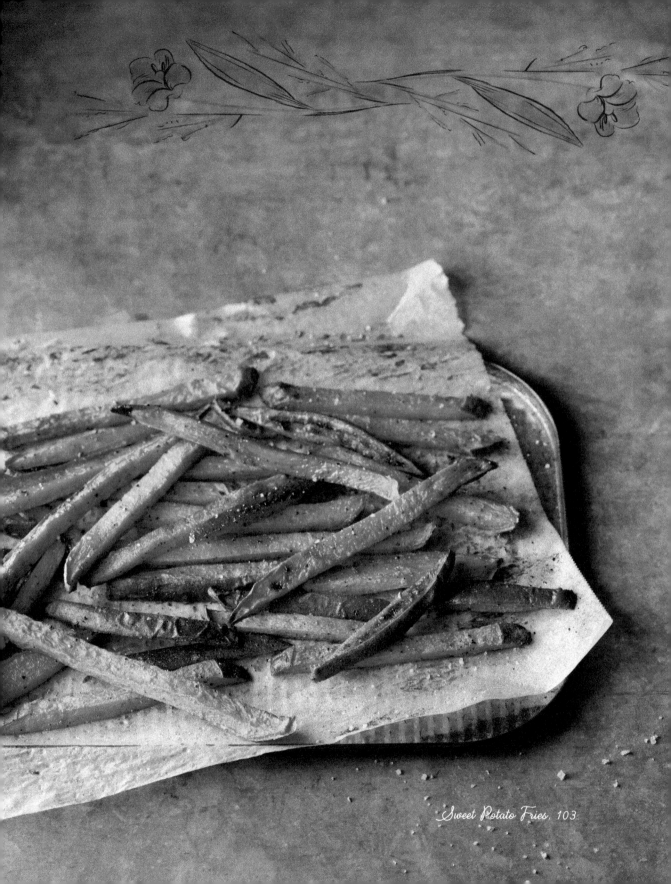

Sweet Potato Fries, 103

CHAPTER SIX

SIDES & SNACKS

Healthy snacks can help fill your nutrient gaps, supply nutrition to your baby throughout the day, regulate your blood sugar and hunger level, and keep your stomach happy and nausea at bay.

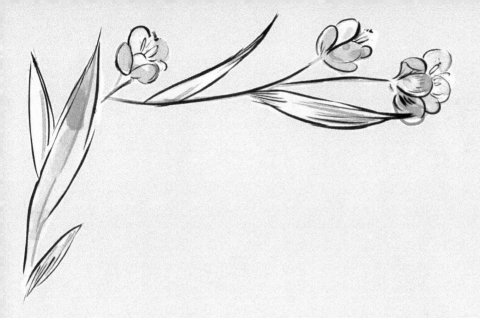

Sides

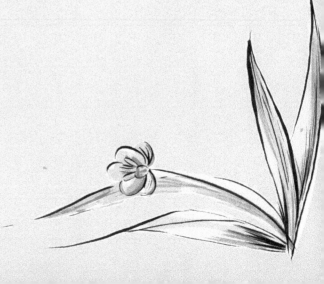

Roasted Potatoes, Carrots, and Asparagus

Prep time: 10 minutes | Cook time: 30 minutes

This recipe is easy to make, and you can add your leftovers to an egg scramble in the morning or your salad at lunch!

Yield: 4 to 5 servings

Serving size: 1 cup

DAIRY-FREE, GLUTEN-FREE,
NUT-FREE, SOY-FREE,
VEGAN, GOOD FOR
CONSTIPATION, GOOD
FOR PRE-CONCEPTION

2 teaspoons dried rosemary

¼ teaspoon salt

¼ teaspoon freshly ground
black pepper

1 pound small purple
potatoes, halved

4 to 5 medium carrots,
cut into ¼-inch rounds

½ tablespoon extra-virgin
olive oil, divided

1 bunch asparagus, cut into
2-inch pieces

Per serving: Calories: 136;
Total fat: 2g; Saturated fat: 0g;
Carbohydrate: 28g; Sugar: 6g;
Fiber: 6g; Protein: 4g; Sodium:
208mg; Cholesterol: 0mg

1. Preheat oven to 425°F.

2. In a small bowl, mix together the rosemary, salt, and pepper.

3. Spread out the carrots and potatoes evenly on a baking sheet. Sprinkle ¼ tablespoon of the oil on the veggies and all of the seasoning mixture.

4. Roast the carrots and potatoes in the oven for 15 minutes.

5. Add the asparagus to the baking sheet with the carrots and potatoes and sprinkle with the remaining ¼ tablespoon of oil.

6. Bake for an additional 15 minutes, or until the potatoes are brown and crisp on the edges.

Tip: Combine this side with the Baked Chicken Legs recipe (page 79) to complete your weeknight dinner. Double both recipes and use the leftovers for lunches during the week.

Roasted Broccoli with Shallots

Prep time: 5 minutes | Cook time: 20 minutes

Shallots are a part of the onion family and a close relation to garlic, which means they are packed with flavor. They are really great in combination with other vegetables and in sauces or dressings.

Yield: 4 servings

Serving size: 1 cup

DAIRY-FREE, GLUTEN-FREE, NUT-FREE, SOY-FREE, VEGAN, GESTATIONAL DIABETES–FRIENDLY, GOOD FOR CONSTIPATION, QUICK

1 broccoli head, cut into florets

1 medium shallot, diced

1 tablespoon extra-virgin olive oil

½ teaspoon salt

½ teaspoon freshly ground black pepper

1. Preheat the oven to 375°F.

2. Spread out the broccoli and shallot evenly on a baking sheet.

3. Sprinkle the oil, salt, and pepper on top of the veggies. Push the veggies around on the baking sheet with a spatula to coat everything well.

4. Roast in the oven for approximately 20 minutes.

Per serving: Calories: 63; Total fat: 4g; Saturated fat: 1g; Carbohydrate: 7g; Sugar: 2g; Fiber: 2g; Protein: 3g; Sodium: 321mg; Cholesterol: 0mg

Sweet Potato Fries

Prep time: 10 to 40 minutes | Cook time: 30 minutes

Avocado oil has a high smoke point and is good to use when you are cooking at higher temperatures, as in this recipe. It also increases your absorption of the fat-soluble nutrients in the sweet potatoes (vitamins A, D, E, and K).

Yield: 4 servings
Serving size: ¾ cup

DAIRY-FREE, GLUTEN-FREE, NUT-FREE, SOY-FREE, VEGAN, GOOD FOR POST-PARTUM RECOVERY, KID-FRIENDLY

2 small to medium sweet potatoes, cut into 3-inch spears
1 teaspoon salt
1 teaspoon freshly ground black pepper
1 teaspoon garlic powder
2 tablespoons avocado oil

Per serving: Calories: 121; Total fat: 7g; Saturated fat: 1g; Carbohydrate: 14g; Sugar: 3g; Fiber: 2g; Protein: 1g; Sodium: 618mg; Cholesterol: 0mg

1. Preheat the oven to 425°F. Line a baking sheet with parchment paper and set aside.

2. Fill a large mixing bowl with cold water, add the potato spears, and allow them to soak for 30 minutes. This reduces the starch content of the potatoes, allowing them to crisp up when baked. (You can skip this step if you're short on time.)

3. If you soaked the potatoes, drain the water and dry them with a paper towel. Add the salt, pepper, garlic powder, and oil to the bowl and toss to coat the potatoes.

4. Spread the fries out evenly on the prepared baking sheet, making sure they aren't overlapping each other, if possible.

5. Bake for 15 minutes. Remove the baking sheet from the oven and flip the potatoes. Bake for an additional 15 minutes, or until you notice the fries turning brown on the edges.

Tip: If you want to enjoy leftover fries with another meal, toast them in a toaster oven or put them under the broiler for a few minutes to "re-crisp" them.

Shredded Brussels Sprouts, Apples, and Pecans

Prep time: 10 minutes

Brussels sprouts are a cruciferous vegetable loaded with fiber, potassium, and vitamins K and C.

Yield: 8 servings

Serving size: ½ cup

DAIRY-FREE, GLUTEN-FREE, SOY-FREE, VEGETARIAN, GOOD FOR CONSTIPATION, GOOD FOR LEG CRAMPS, QUICK

FOR THE SALAD

1 small apple, cored and thinly sliced

3 cups shredded Brussels sprouts

⅓ cup pecans

⅓ cup goat cheese (pasteurized if you are currently pregnant)

FOR THE DRESSING

1 small shallot, chopped

2 tablespoons extra-virgin olive oil

Juice of ½ lemon

2 tablespoons red wine vinegar

¼ teaspoon salt

¼ teaspoon freshly ground black pepper

TO MAKE THE SALAD

Combine the apple, Brussels sprouts, pecans, and cheese in a large bowl.

TO MAKE THE DRESSING

Whisk together all the dressing ingredients and add the dressing to the salad.

Per serving: Calories: 108; Total fat: 8g; Saturated fat: 2g; Carbohydrate: 8g; Sugar: 4g; Fiber: 2g; Protein: 3g; Sodium: 3mg; Cholesterol: 103mg

Parmesan Green Beans and Mushrooms

Prep time: 10 minutes | Cook time: 20 minutes

This one-pan side can be put together in less than 30 minutes. Mushrooms are a great source of copper and selenium. Depending on how they are grown, they can contain vitamin D, which is a rare nutrient to find in whole foods.

Yield: 6 servings
Serving size: 1 cup

GLUTEN-FREE, NUT-FREE, SOY-FREE, VEGETARIAN, GESTATIONAL DIABETES-FRIENDLY, QUICK

1 pound fresh green beans
10 ounces mushrooms, sliced
4 garlic cloves, minced
2 tablespoons extra-virgin olive oil
½ teaspoon salt
¼ teaspoon freshly ground black pepper
3 tablespoons Parmesan cheese

Per serving: Calories: 138; Total fat: 9g; Saturated fat: 2g; Carbohydrate: 12g; Sugar: 3g; Fiber: 5g; Protein: 7g; Sodium: 367mg; Cholesterol: 5mg

1. Preheat the oven to 375°F.

2. Spread out the green beans and mushrooms evenly on a large baking sheet. It doesn't matter if they are overlapping.

3. Scatter the garlic evenly over the veggies.

4. Sprinkle everything with the oil, salt, and pepper.

5. Use a spatula to mix the veggies, coating them evenly in the oil and spices.

6. Bake for around 20 minutes. Remove from the oven and sprinkle on the Parmesan cheese before serving.

Tip: This side pairs well with Almond-Crusted Cod (page 81). Leave off the cheese to make this recipe dairy-free.

Simple Coleslaw

Prep time: 10 minutes

This easy-to-make dish is great to bring to a barbecue.

Yield: 6 to 8 servings
Serving size: ½ cup

GLUTEN-FREE, NUT-FREE,
SOY-FREE, VEGETARIAN,
GOOD FOR CONSTIPATION,
QUICK

1 teaspoon Dijon mustard
5 tablespoons mayonnaise
1 tablespoon apple
   cider vinegar
¼ teaspoon onion powder
1 teaspoon sugar
¼ cup Greek yogurt, any
   fat level
6 cups shredded cabbage
   and carrots
Salt, for seasoning
Freshly ground black pepper,
   for seasoning

Per serving: Calories: 103; Total
fat: 9g; Saturated fat: 1g; Carbohydrate: 5g; Sugar: 3g; Fiber:
2g; Protein: 2g; Sodium: 128mg;
Cholesterol: 5mg

1. In a small bowl, combine the mustard, mayon-naise, vinegar, onion powder, sugar, and yogurt.

2. In a large bowl, add the cabbage and carrots.

3. Add the dressing to the cabbage and carrots and mix well. Season with salt and pepper.

Tip: Pair this side with Slow-Cooked Pulled Pork (page 77).

THREE-GRAIN ANCIENT BLEND

Prep time: 5 minutes | Cook time: 30 minutes

You can prepare this recipe as a side dish or as a breakfast like oatmeal! Get out of your comfort zone a bit and try these ancient grains.

Yield: 3 servings

Serving size: ¾ cup

DAIRY-FREE, GLUTEN-FREE, NUT-FREE, SOY-FREE, VEGAN, GOOD FOR POSTPARTUM RECOVERY

3 cups vegetable broth

⅓ cup uncooked teff

⅓ cup uncooked millet

⅓ cup uncooked amaranth

Per serving: Calories: 239; Total fat: 4g; Saturated fat: 1g; Carbohydrate: 39g; Sugar: 1g; Fiber: 5g; Protein: 12g; Sodium: 771mg; Cholesterol: 0mg

1. Bring the broth to a boil in a medium pot over high heat.

2. Add teff, millet, and amaranth, cover the pot, and reduce the heat to medium-low.

3. Let simmer for 20 to 25 minutes, or until all the broth has been absorbed. Fluff the cooked grains with a fork before serving.

Tip: If you are using this dish as your morning oatmeal, use water instead of broth and add milk once it's done cooking. Top with your favorite oatmeal toppings.

CAULIFLOWER MASH

Prep time: 10 minutes | Cook time: 10 minutes

I don't recommend replacing all your carbs with cauliflower, but it is a great alternative if you are struggling with high blood sugar. Plus, cauliflower offers a ton of nutrients.

Yield: 4 servings
Serving size: ½ cup

GLUTEN-FREE, NUT-FREE,
SOY-FREE, VEGETARIAN,
GESTATIONAL DIABETES–
FRIENDLY, GOOD FOR
POSTPARTUM RECOVERY

1 cauliflower head,
   cut into large chunks
1 tablespoon extra-virgin
   olive oil
1 teaspoon minced garlic
1 tablespoon butter
1 teaspoon salt
½ teaspoon freshly ground
   black pepper
1 teaspoon chopped chives
1 teaspoon chopped flat
   leaf parsley

Per serving: Calories: 93;
Total fat: 7g; Saturated fat: 2g;
Carbohydrate: 8g; Sugar: 4g;
Fiber: 4g; Protein: 3g; Sodium:
645mg; Cholesterol: 8mg

1. Steam the cauliflower in an Instant Pot® or steamer basket on the stove for 6 to 8 minutes, or until the cauliflower is tender.

2. While the cauliflower is steaming, heat the oil in a small skillet over medium heat and sauté the garlic for 1 or 2 minutes.

3. Transfer the steamed cauliflower to a large mixing bowl. Add the garlic, butter, salt, and pepper. Mash the cauliflower with a potato masher, hand mixer, or immersion blender.

4. Stir in the chives and parsley before serving.

Tip: Avoid boiling the cauliflower, as it will hold too much water. This side dish would pair well with Pan-Seared Rainbow Trout (page 90).

FRESH VEGGIE COUSCOUS

Prep time: 15 minutes | Cook time: 10 minutes

The Israeli couscous in this recipe is a bit larger than average couscous, is toasted rather than dried, and has a chewier, more pasta-like taste. You could include this delicious side dish with your work lunches all week. It pairs nicely with fish, lamb, or chicken.

Yield: 8 servings
Serving size: 1 cup

DAIRY-FREE, NUT-FREE, SOY-FREE, VEGAN, GOOD FOR CONSTIPATION, GOOD FOR PRE-CONCEPTION, QUICK

1½ cups dried Israeli couscous

1 (15.5-ounce) can chickpeas, drained and rinsed

1 medium English cucumber, diced

1 large tomato, diced

¼ cup extra-virgin olive oil

1 teaspoon Dijon mustard

½ teaspoon honey

2 tablespoons fresh squeezed lemon juice

1 teaspoon lemon zest

½ teaspoon sea salt

¼ teaspoon freshly ground black pepper

½ cup coarsely chopped fresh basil

½ cup coarsely chopped fresh parsley

Per serving: Calories: 263; Total fat: 7g; Saturated fat: 1g; Carbohydrate: 42g; Sugar: 2g; Fiber: 5g; Protein: 8g; Sodium: 311mg; Cholesterol: 0mg

1. Bring a large pot of water to a boil over high heat and add the couscous. Reduce the heat to low, cover the pot, and cook for about 8 minutes. Drain the water from the couscous and set the couscous aside.

2. In a large bowl, combine the chickpeas, cucumber, and tomato.

3. In a small bowl, combine the oil, mustard, honey, lemon juice, lemon zest, salt, and pepper.

4. Add the couscous and dressing to the large bowl and toss everything together.

5. Sprinkle the basil and parsley on top and enjoy warm or cold.

Tip: Gluten-free couscous is available. Look for it at your local store if you have a sensitivity.

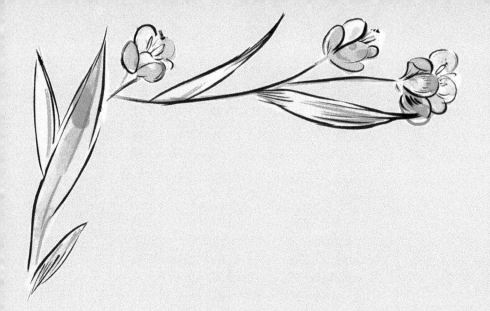

Snacks

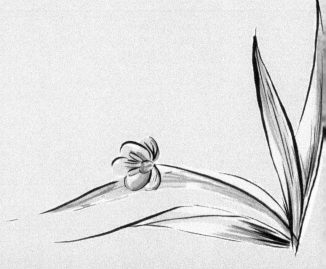

TURMERIC HUMMUS

Prep time: 10 minutes

Hummus is very easy to make at home. Most of the ingredients in this recipe are what I consider pantry staples, so you likely won't even need to make a trip to the store.

Yield: 12 servings

Serving size:

2 tablespoons

DAIRY-FREE, GLUTEN-FREE, NUT-FREE, SOY-FREE, VEGAN, GOOD FOR PRE-CONCEPTION, QUICK

1 (15.5-ounce) can chickpeas, drained and rinsed

2 tablespoons extra-virgin olive oil

1 tablespoon lemon juice

4 garlic cloves

½ teaspoon turmeric

¼ teaspoon salt

¼ teaspoon freshly ground black pepper

Per serving: Calories: 70; Total fat: 3g; Saturated fat: 0g; Carbohydrate: 10g; Sugar: 0g; Fiber: 2g; Protein: 2g; Sodium: 170mg; Cholesterol: 0mg

Add all the ingredients to a food processor and blend until the hummus is a creamy consistency.

Tip: Enjoy this dip with fresh veggies like colorful bell peppers, carrots, and cherry tomatoes.

Peanut Butter Energy Bites

Prep time: 10 minutes

Women often struggle with sweet cravings during pregnancy. This recipe will help satisfy your afternoon sweet tooth.

Yield: 6 to 12 servings

Serving size: 1 to 2 balls

GLUTEN-FREE, SOY-FREE, VEGETARIAN, ENERGY ENHANCER, GOOD FOR LACTATION, KID-FRIENDLY

1 cup gluten-free old-fashioned rolled oats

½ cup ground flaxseed or flaxseed meal

½ cup peanut butter

½ cup dark chocolate chips

2 tablespoons chia seeds

¼ cup maple syrup

⅓ cup unsweetened coconut flakes (optional)

Per serving: Calories: 333; Total fat: 19g; Saturated fat: 5g; Carbohydrate: 34g; Sugar: 15g; Fiber: 7g; Protein: 10g; Sodium: 104mg; Cholesterol: 0mg

1. Combine all the ingredients in a large mixing bowl.

2. Form into 1-inch balls.

3. Store in an air-tight container in the refrigerator.

Tip: Chocolate chips aren't always dairy-free, so be sure to read the package label if you have a dairy allergy. Similarly, oats are often processed in plants that also process products with gluten. If you have celiac disease or are sensitive to gluten, ensure the label states the oats are gluten-free.

Berry Parfait

Prep time: 5 minutes

This parfait is one of my go-to snacks. Granola and fruit-flavored yogurt often have a lot of added sugar. Buy plain yogurt and add your own sweetener and berries. Frozen berries tend to be more sweet than fresh because of the juices they release when they thaw.

Yield: 1 serving

Serving size: 4 ounces of yogurt and toppings

GLUTEN-FREE, SOY-FREE, VEGETARIAN, GOOD FOR CONSTIPATION, GOOD FOR PRE-CONCEPTION, QUICK

4 ounces plain Greek yogurt

1 teaspoon stevia

¾ cup fresh berries (blueberries, raspberries, blackberries)

2 teaspoons chia seeds

1 tablespoon slivered almonds

1 tablespoon coconut flakes, unsweetened

Per serving: Calories: 236; Total fat: 9g; Saturated fat: 3g; Carbohydrate: 26g; Sugar: 15g; Fiber: 7g; Protein: 15g; Sodium: 53mg; Cholesterol: 10mg

1. In a medium bowl, mix together the yogurt and stevia.

2. Fold the berries, chia seeds, almonds, and coconut into the yogurt.

Tip: To make this recipe dairy-free, choose a coconut- or cashew-based yogurt, but understand these varieties will not be a good source of protein, B vitamins, iodine, or vitamin K.

Roasted Chickpeas

Prep time: 5 minutes | Cook time: 30 minutes

Roasted chickpeas can add a nice crunch to salads and a little extra protein if you are vegetarian. They are a good snack during the first trimester because of their folate content.

Yield: 6 servings

Serving size: ¼ cup

DAIRY-FREE, GLUTEN-FREE, NUT-FREE, SOY-FREE, VEGAN, GOOD FOR POSTPARTUM RECOVERY

1 (15.5-ounce) can chickpeas, drained and rinsed

1 tablespoon extra-virgin olive oil

¾ teaspoon garlic powder

½ teaspoon Italian seasoning

½ teaspoon salt

½ teaspoon freshly ground black pepper

1. Preheat oven to 375°F.

2. Spread the chickpeas out evenly on a large rimmed baking sheet.

3. Roast for 30 minutes, opening the oven a few times to shake the baking sheet to rotate the chickpeas.

4. As the chickpeas roast, mix together the oil, garlic powder, Italian seasoning, salt, and pepper in a large bowl.

5. Add the roasted chickpeas to the seasoning mixture and stir thoroughly to coat them.

Per serving: Calories: 118; Total fat: 3g; Saturated fat: 0g; Carbohydrate: 19g; Sugar: 0g; Fiber: 4g; Protein: 4g; Sodium: 433mg; Cholesterol: 0mg

Citrus Snack Plate

Prep time: 12 minutes

Did you know that avocados are a fruit? They are the state fruit in my home state of California, and we pretty much add them to everything. This dish has loads of vitamin C, fiber, antioxidants, and so many other nutrients.

Yield: 2 to 3 servings

Serving size: 1 cup

DAIRY-FREE, GLUTEN-FREE, NUT-FREE, SOY-FREE, VEGAN, GOOD FOR CONSTIPATION, GOOD FOR PRE-CONCEPTION, QUICK

FOR THE SALAD

2 cups arugula

2 small Cara Cara oranges, peeled and cut into ¼-inch slices

1 grapefruit, peeled and cut into ¼-inch slices

1 medium avocado, peeled, pitted, and cut into ¼-inch slices

½ cup pomegranate seeds

FOR THE DRESSING

½ shallot, diced

1 tablespoon white wine vinegar

½ cup extra-virgin olive oil

Juice of ½ lemon

½ teaspoon lemon zest

1 tablespoon fresh thyme

Pinch salt

Pinch freshly ground black pepper

TO MAKE THE SALAD

Arrange the arugula on a plate and top it with the oranges, grapefruit, avocado, and pomegranate.

TO MAKE THE DRESSING

Whisk together the dressing ingredients and drizzle over the plate of colorful fruit.

Per serving: Calories: 726; Total fat: 64g; Saturated fat: 9g; Carbohydrate: 43g; Sugar: 26g; Fiber: 12g; Protein: 5g; Sodium: 18mg; Cholesterol: 0mg

Mozzarella Bites

Prep time: 10 minutes | Cook time: 5 to 7 minutes

Almond meal is ground almonds, but it's not fine enough to be considered a flour. It's the perfect substitute for bread crumbs. Because these mozzarella bites are made with almond meal, they are relatively low in carbs and are gestational diabetes-friendly.

Yield: 5 servings
Serving size: 4 bites

GLUTEN-FREE, SOY-FREE, VEGETARIAN, GESTATIONAL DIABETES–FRIENDLY, GOOD FOR POSTPARTUM RECOVERY, KID-FRIENDLY, QUICK

Olive oil spray
1 large egg
½ cup almond meal
¼ teaspoon garlic powder
4 mozzarella cheese sticks, cut into fifths
½ cup marinara sauce (optional)

Per serving: Calories: 133; Total fat: 10g; Saturated fat: 3g; Carbohydrate: 3g; Sugar: 1g; Fiber: 1g; Protein: 10g; Sodium: 148mg; Cholesterol: 45mg

1. Preheat the oven to 350°F. Spray a baking sheet with oil and set aside.

2. In a small bowl whisk the egg.

3. In a medium bowl, combine the almond meal and garlic powder.

4. Dip the cheese pieces in the egg and then sprinkle them all over with the almond meal mixture (see Tip).

5. Place each piece of cheese on the oiled baking sheet.

6. Bake for 5 to 7 minutes, watching carefully so the cheese sticks don't melt completely.

7. Enjoy with a marinara sauce dip, if desired.

Tip: The almond meal coagulates quickly when it comes in contact with the egg. Instead of dropping the cheese pieces into the almond meal, hold them in one hand while you sprinkle the almond meal onto the cheese with your other hand.

Traditional Caprese Salad

Prep time: 15 minutes | Cook time: 10 minutes

This low-carb snack also makes a delicious appetizer, though you might want to avoid it if you are experiencing a lot of heartburn.

Yield: 4 servings
Serving size: 1 cup

GLUTEN-FREE, NUT-FREE, SOY-FREE, VEGETARIAN, GESTATIONAL DIABETES–FRIENDLY, QUICK

10 ounces cherry tomatoes

¼ cup chopped fresh basil

½ teaspoon sea salt

¼ teaspoon freshly ground pepper

1 tablespoon extra-virgin olive oil

½ cup balsamic vinegar

1½ tablespoons honey

8 ounces fresh mozzarella cheese

Per serving: Calories: 234; Total fat: 16g; Saturated fat: 1g; Carbohydrate: 12g; Sugar: 9g; Fiber: 1g; Protein: 11g; Sodium: 279mg; Cholesterol: 40mg

1. Add the tomatoes, basil, salt, pepper, and oil to a large bowl.

2. Heat the balsamic vinegar and honey in a small skillet over medium heat until the mixture bubbles. Reduce the heat to low and let the mixture thicken, 8 to 10 minutes. Remove the mixture from the heat immediately once it thickens.

3. Meanwhile, use a tablespoon to scoop balls of the mozzarella cheese into the bowl with the tomato mixture.

4. Once the balsamic glaze is done, add it slowly to the large bowl and toss the ingredients together.

Tip: If you aren't looking for something low carb, this salad would be great with focaccia or fried bread.

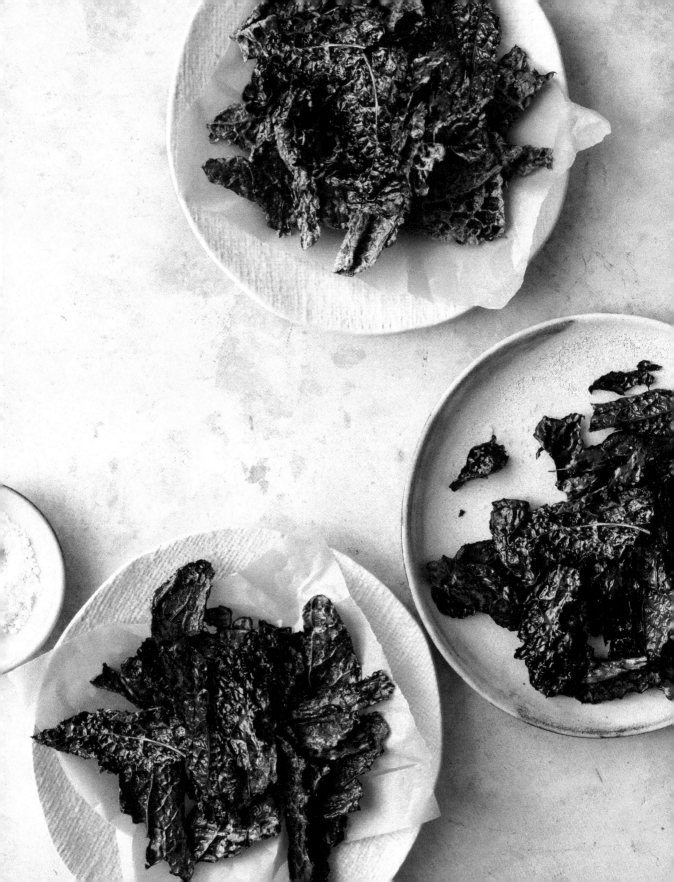

Home-Baked Kale Chips

Prep time: 10 minutes | Cook time: 10 to 12 minutes

Kale chips are the perfect snack if you are craving something crunchy and salty. They may not always satisfy your craving for chips, but they are a great alternative to traditional snack foods filled with empty calories.

Yield: 2 servings
Serving size: 1 cup

DAIRY-FREE, GLUTEN-FREE, NUT-FREE, SOY-FREE, VEGAN, GESTATIONAL DIABETES–FRIENDLY, QUICK

1 bunch kale, torn into bite-size pieces

1 tablespoon extra-virgin olive oil

1 teaspoon garlic salt

1. Preheat the oven to 350°F. Line a baking sheet with parchment paper and set aside.

2. Place the kale pieces in a large mixing bowl and toss with oil and garlic salt.

3. Spread the kale out in an even layer on the prepared baking sheet.

4. Bake for 10 to 12 minutes.

Per serving: Calories: 131; Total fat: 7g; Saturated fat: 1g; Carbohydrate: 15g; Sugar: 0g; Fiber: 2g; Protein: 4g; Sodium: 58mg; Cholesterol: 0mg

Artichoke, Spinach, and White Bean Dip

Prep time: 10 minutes | Cook time: 15 minutes

This twist on classic spinach and artichoke dip is a great appetizer or snack option. White beans add fiber, protein, and other nutrients. The beans also add carbs, a consideration if you have gestational diabetes.

Yield: 8 servings

Serving size: ¼ cup

GLUTEN-FREE, NUT-FREE, SOY-FREE, VEGETARIAN, GOOD FOR PRE-CONCEPTION, QUICK

1 teaspoon extra-virgin olive oil

2 garlic cloves, minced

2 cups fresh spinach

¾ cup white beans

8 ounces cream cheese

1 (14-ounce) can artichoke hearts, drained

1 cup Parmesan cheese

1 teaspoon dried basil

1 teaspoon dried oregano

¼ teaspoon salt

2 teaspoons freshly squeezed lemon juice

1. Preheat the oven to 350°F.

2. Heat the oil in a medium skillet over medium heat and sauté the garlic and spinach for 2 to 3 minutes.

3. In a food processor, add the beans and cream cheese. Blend until smooth.

4. Add the artichokes, Parmesan cheese, basil, oregano, salt, and lemon juice and pulse.

5. Remove the mixture from the food processor and place it in an oven-safe dish. Stir in the spinach and garlic mixture. Bake uncovered for 15 minutes.

6. Enjoy with pita chips, tortilla chips, or veggies.

Per serving: Calories: 199; Total fat: 14g; Saturated fat: 8g; Carbohydrate: 11g; Sugar: 1g; Fiber: 4g; Protein: 10g; Sodium: 341mg; Cholesterol: 41mg

CLASSIC DEVILED EGGS

Prep time: 10 minutes

These eggs are a great appetizer or party snack, and you can even enjoy them for breakfast!

Yield: 6 servings

Serving size:

2 deviled eggs

GLUTEN-FREE, NUT-FREE, SOY-FREE, VEGETARIAN, GOOD FOR PRE-CONCEPTION, KID-FRIENDLY, QUICK

6 hardboiled eggs, peeled and halved

3 tablespoons mayonnaise

1 tablespoon yellow mustard

1 teaspoon vinegar

Pinch salt

1 teaspoon paprika, optional

1. Separate the egg yolks from the whites. Place the yolks in a small mixing bowl and the whites on a plate.

2. To the bowl with the yolks, add the mayo, mustard, vinegar, and salt and stir until the mixture is smooth and creamy.

3. Fill each egg white with the yolk mixture and sprinkle with paprika, if desired.

Per serving: Calories: 110; Total fat: 10g; Saturated fat: 2g; Carbohydrate: 1g; Sugar: 0g; Fiber: 0g; Protein: 6g; Sodium: 174mg; Cholesterol: 166mg

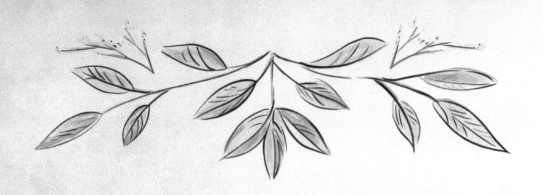

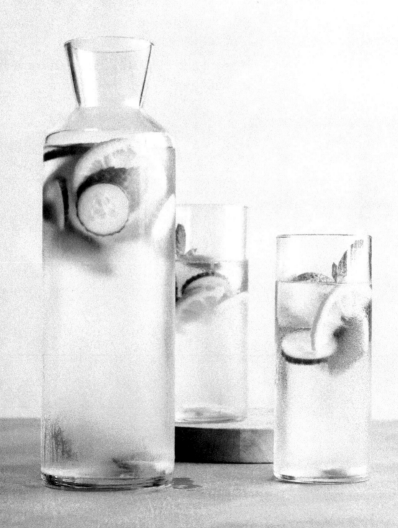

Knockout Nausea Water. 125

CHAPTER SEVEN

DRINKS & DESSERTS

If you're like me, you agree that dessert is the best part of any meal. Dessert may not provide us with as much nutrition as breakfast, salads, or soups, but a little sweetness does provide us with pleasure and joy. This chapter includes delicious drinks that double as practical remedies for curbing nausea or boosting lactation.

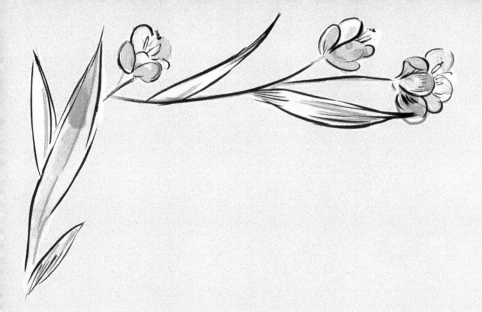

Drinks

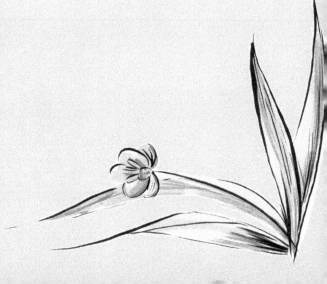

KNOCKOUT NAUSEA WATER

Prep time: 10 minutes

Nausea can be a real bummer in and sometimes beyond the first trimester. Ginger has been used for decades to help alleviate upset stomachs. It's safe for all and effective for most.

Yield: 8 servings

Serving size: 8 ounces

DAIRY-FREE, GLUTEN-FREE, NUT-FREE, SOY-FREE, VEGAN, GOOD FOR NAUSEA, GOOD FOR POST-PARTUM RECOVERY

2 liters filtered water
2 lemons, thinly sliced
½ large seedless cucumber, thinly sliced
1 teaspoon grated fresh ginger
8 mint leaves

1. Pour the water into a 2-liter pitcher or carafe.

2. Add the lemon, cucumber, ginger, and mint to the water.

3. The water will keep in the refrigerator for up to 5 days.

Per serving: Calories: 8; Total fat: 0g; Saturated fat: 0g; Carbohydrate: 2g; Sugar: 1g; Fiber: 1g; Protein: 0g; Sodium: 2mg; Cholesterol: 0mg

BERRY- AND BASIL-INFUSED WATER

Prep time: 10 minutes

Do you have a hard time drinking enough water throughout the day? If you get bored with plain water, try this infused version to add some healthy flavor!

Yield: 4 servings

Serving size: 8 ounces

DAIRY-FREE, GLUTEN-FREE, NUT-FREE, SOY-FREE, VEGAN, GOOD FOR POST-PARTUM RECOVERY, GOOD FOR SWELLING, QUICK

1 quart filtered water
1 cup sliced strawberries
1 cup blueberries
1 handful fresh basil

1. Pour the water into a 1-liter pitcher or carafe.

2. Add the strawberries, blueberries, and basil to the water.

3. The water will keep in the refrigerator for up to 5 days.

Per serving: Calories: 5; Total fat: 0g; Saturated fat: 0g; Carbohydrate: 1g; Sugar: 1g; Fiber: 0g; Protein: 0g; Sodium: 0mg; Cholesterol: 0mg

ELECTROLYTE BALANCE

Prep time: 10 minutes

If you've actually been vomiting, I recommend making this drink. Sports drinks that provide electrolytes are often made with a lot of unnecessary sugar. Use this recipe instead if you are feeling dehydrated.

Yield: 4 servings
Serving size: 8 ounces

DAIRY-FREE, GLUTEN-FREE, NUT-FREE, SOY-FREE, VEGAN, GOOD FOR LEG CRAMPS, GOOD FOR NAUSEA, GOOD FOR SWELLING, MAY HELP WITH HEADACHES

Juice of 1 lemon
½ cup 100 percent apple juice or orange juice
¼ teaspoon salt
½ teaspoon stevia
1 liter coconut water, unsweetened

1. In a medium pitcher or carafe, add the lemon juice, fruit juice, salt, and stevia.

2. Add the coconut water and stir everything together.

Per serving: Calories: 159; Total fat: 0g; Saturated fat: 0g; Carbohydrate: 39g; Sugar: 39g; Fiber: 0g; Protein: 0g; Sodium: 180mg; Cholesterol: 0mg

Caffeine-Free Vanilla Latte

Prep time: 7 minutes

There are a lot of coffee alternatives, such as maca powder, mushroom coffee, chai blends, Dandy Blend, etc. Having an alternative is a good idea if you consume more than one cup of coffee per day.

Yield: 1 serving

Serving size: 12 ounces

DAIRY-FREE, GLUTEN-FREE, SOY-FREE, QUICK

1 cup almond milk

½ cup coconut milk

¼ teaspoon vanilla extract

1 scoop collagen peptides

Combine all the ingredients in a microwave-safe mug and warm in the microwave for 1 minute. An alternative preparation is to heat the ingredients in a small pot on the stove for a few minutes.

Per serving: Calories: 360; Total fat: 35g; Saturated fat: 25g; Carbohydrate: 9g; Sugar: 4g; Fiber: 5g; Protein: 5g; Sodium: 378mg; Cholesterol: 0mg

LACTATION TEA BLEND

Prep time: 10 minutes | Cook time: 10 minutes

There is no concrete scientific evidence that lactation teas increase your milk supply, but some women find they work well for them. Chamomile tea may not only increase milk supply but also promote relaxation, improve sleep, and reduce anxiety.

Yield: 6 servings, ¾ cup loose leaf tea

Serving size: 8 ounces, 2 tablespoons loose leaf tea

DAIRY-FREE, GLUTEN-FREE, SOY-FREE, VEGAN, GOOD FOR LACTATION, GOOD FOR POSTPARTUM RECOVERY

¼ cup fenugreek seeds
¼ cup dried blessed thistle
¼ cup loose leaf
   chamomile flowers

Per serving: Calories: 0; Total fat: 0g; Saturated fat: 0g; Carbohydrate: 0g; Sugar: 0g; Fiber: 0g; Protein: 0g; Sodium: 0mg; Cholesterol: 0mg

1. Combine all three herbs in a glass jar.
2. Boil 8 ounces of water.
3. Scoop 2 tablespoons of the herb blend into a loose leaf tea-diffusing pouch.
4. Once the water is boiling, add it to a mug and place the tea-diffusing pouch in the hot water to steep for 2 to 3 minutes.

Tip: Buy USDA-certified organic, fair trade tea. It's the best way to ensure you're consuming quality products. Teas and herbals aren't tightly regulated, so they have a higher chance of containing heavy metals or environmental pollutants.

Sugar-Free Freshly Squeezed Lemonade

Prep time: 10 minutes

This is a great drink for hot summer days. As far as sugar alternatives go, stevia is the best option. It is a lot sweeter than table sugar, so you don't need to use as much.

Yield: 2 servings

Serving size: 8 ounces

DAIRY-FREE, GLUTEN-FREE, NUT-FREE, SOY-FREE, VEGAN, GESTATIONAL DIABETES–FRIENDLY, KID-FRIENDLY, QUICK

¼ cup freshly squeezed lemon juice

2 tablespoons stevia

2 cups filtered water

Add the lemon juice and stevia to 2 cups water and stir together.

Per serving: Calories: 7; Total fat: 0g; Saturated fat: 0g; Carbohydrate: 1g; Sugar: 1g; Fiber: 0g; Protein: 0g; Sodium: 6mg; Cholesterol: 0mg

PINEAPPLE MOJITO MOCKTAIL

Prep time: 10 minutes

If you are feeling left out of the party when everyone else is drinking, try this mocktail!

Yield: 2 servings

Serving size: 1 cup

DAIRY-FREE, GLUTEN-FREE, NUT-FREE, SOY-FREE, VEGETARIAN, QUICK

12 mint leaves

4 tablespoons honey

¼ cup freshly squeezed lime juice

½ cup pineapple juice

2 cups sparkling water

1. Divide the mint leaves, honey, and lime juice between 2 glasses.

2. Use a wooden spoon to gently muddle the mint leaves while mixing together the other ingredients. Divide the pineapple juice between each glass.

3. Fill each glass with ice and then add 1 cup of sparkling water.

Per serving: Calories: 177; Total fat: 0g; Saturated fat: 0g; Carbohydrate: 47g; Sugar: 42g; Fiber: 2g; Protein: 1g; Sodium: 10mg; Cholesterol: 0mg

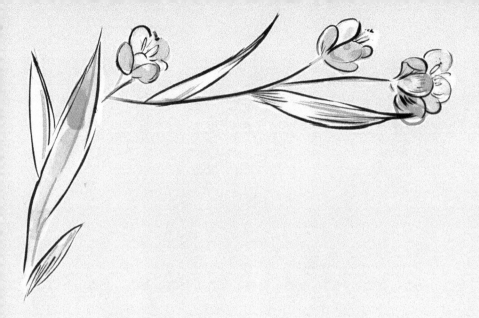

Desserts

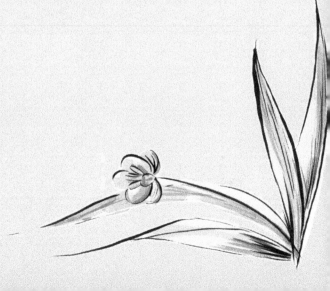

STRAWBERRIES AND CREAM

Prep time: 10 minutes

I love whipped cream, and I also love the fact that it is super easy to make at home. It tastes better and doesn't have any unnecessary ingredients like the store-bought versions do. That's what I call a win-win-win!

Yield: 2 cups whipped cream (4 servings)

Serving size: ¼ cup whipped cream and ½ cup strawberries

GLUTEN-FREE, NUT-FREE, SOY-FREE, VEGETARIAN, QUICK

8 ounces heavy
    whipping cream
1 tablespoon stevia
1 tablespoon vanilla extract
2 cups sliced strawberries

Per serving: Calories: 113; Total fat: 11g; Saturated fat: 7g; Carbohydrate: 2g; Sugar: 1g; Fiber: 0g; Protein: 1g; Sodium: 12mg; Cholesterol: 41mg

1. If possible, place your mixing bowl in the freezer for 10 minutes prior to whipping the cream to help it thicken faster.

2. Place the heavy whipping cream, stevia, and vanilla in the bowl.

3. Whip on medium to high speed until the cream becomes thick.

4. Place a dollop of whipped cream on top of the strawberries.

Tip: Use this whipped cream to top the Blueberry Pecan Pancakes (page 28)!

DARK CHOCOLATE–COVERED RAISINS

Prep time: 10 minutes | Cook time: 1 to 2 minutes

This is what I consider a "healthy" dessert. (I add quotation marks because these raisins do contain a decent amount of sugar!) Did you know dark chocolate is a good source of magnesium? Raisins also provide fiber, potassium, and antioxidants.

Yield: 2 cups

Serving size: ¼ cup

GLUTEN-FREE, NUT-FREE, SOY-FREE, KID-FRIENDLY, QUICK

8 ounces dark chocolate, broken up into pieces

8 ounces seedless raisins

Per serving: Calories: 209; Total fat: 8g; Saturated fat: 6g; Carbohydrate: 40g; Sugar: 31g; Fiber: 3g; Protein: 2g; Sodium: 13mg; Cholesterol: 1mg

1. Cover two dinner plates with parchment paper.

2. Place the chocolate in a glass bowl. Microwave for 1 to 2 minutes or until the chocolate is fully melted.

3. Cover the raisins in the chocolate and place them on the prepared plates in an even layer.

4. Chill the raisins in the refrigerator or freezer for 20 minutes for faster hardening. Enjoy once the chocolate has hardened.

Tip: It may be a bit messy dipping the raisins, but that also makes it fun. If you have kids, you can get them involved, too. The next time you go to the movies, pack up a small bag to snack on in the theater!

Cinnamon Sugar Apples

Prep time: 10 minutes | Cook time: 40 minutes

My mouth is watering just thinking about this dish. The lack of crust means this apple dessert is relatively low in carbs.

Yield: 4 servings

Serving size: 1 half apple

GLUTEN-FREE, SOY-FREE, VEGETARIAN

1 tablespoon ground cinnamon

1 tablespoon sugar

2 tablespoons butter, preferably grass-fed

2 medium apples, cored and halved

2 tablespoons chopped walnuts

1. Preheat the oven to 400°F.

2. Combine the cinnamon and sugar in a small microwavable bowl. Place the butter on top and melt it in the microwave for 20 to 30 seconds.

3. Place the apples in a baking pan or on a baking sheet.

4. Sprinkle the walnuts on top of the apples and top with the cinnamon sugar mixture.

5. Bake in the oven for 30 minutes.

6. Serve plain or with a scoop of vanilla ice cream.

Per serving: Calories: 148; Total fat: 8g; Saturated fat: 4g; Carbohydrate: 20g; Sugar: 15g; Fiber: 4g; Protein: 1g; Sodium: 42mg; Cholesterol: 15mg

SEEDY CHOCOLATE BARK

Prep time: 7 minutes | Cooking time: 20 minutes

I love this dessert because you can get creative with different combinations of nuts, seeds, and dried fruit. This recipe will satisfy your sweet tooth while also filling you up with fiber and antioxidants.

Yield: 12 to 15 servings
Serving size: 2-inch square of bark

GLUTEN-FREE, NUT-FREE, SOY-FREE, QUICK

8 ounces dark chocolate, broken up into pieces
¼ cup sunflower seeds
¼ cup pumpkin seeds
1 tablespoon chia seeds
½ cup dried raspberries

1. Cover a 9-by-13-inch glass baking dish with parchment paper.

2. Place the chocolate in a glass bowl. Microwave the chocolate for 1 to 2 minutes, or until fully melted.

3. Spread the chocolate into the prepared baking dish in a thin, even layer.

4. Sprinkle the seeds and raspberries on top.

5. Chill the bark in the refrigerator or freezer for 20 minutes for faster hardening. Once hardened, cut into 2-inch squares for serving.

Per serving: Calories: 116; Total fat: 8g; Saturated fat: 4g; Carbohydrate: 14g; Sugar: 11g; Fiber: 2g; Protein: 2g; Sodium: 8mg; Cholesterol: 1mg

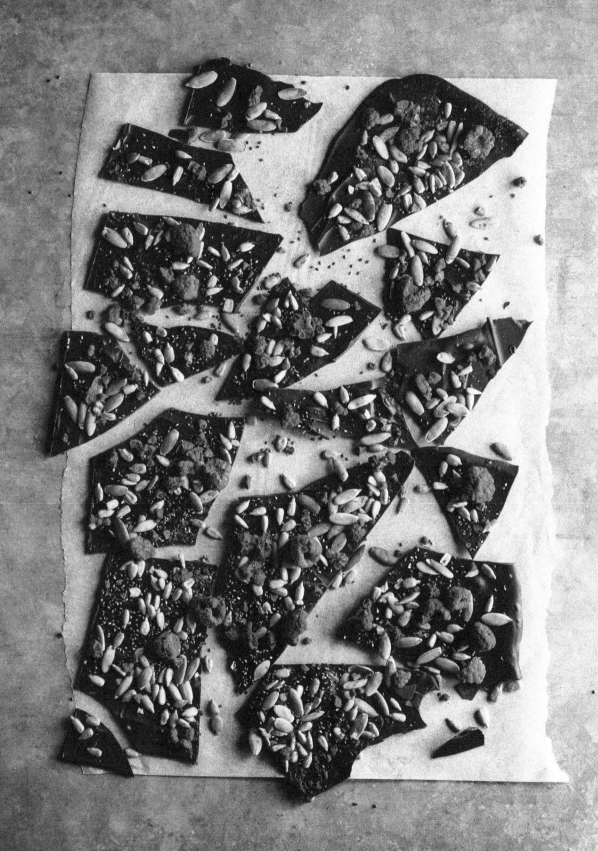

Avocado Chocolate Pudding

You wouldn't know there was avocado in this pudding if you didn't read the recipe. It tastes like chocolate heaven!

Yield: 3 servings

Serving size: ½ cup

GLUTEN-FREE, NUT-FREE, SOY-FREE, VEGETARIAN, GOOD FOR SWELLING, KID-FRIENDLY

1 large avocado, peeled and pitted

¼ cup cocoa powder

1 teaspoon vanilla extract

1 cup heavy whipping cream

3 tablespoons maple syrup

Per serving: Calories: 442; Total fat: 39g; Saturated fat: 20g; Carbohydrate: 25g; Sugar: 13g; Fiber: 6g; Protein: 4g; Sodium: 38mg; Cholesterol: 109mg

1. Place all the ingredients in a large mixing bowl.

2. Using a standing mixer or hand mixer, beat on high speed for about 3 minutes until the mixture develops a pudding consistency.

Tip: Enjoy this pudding the day you make it or the day after.

Mini Blueberry Pies

Prep time: 10 minutes | Cook time: 20 minutes

I love these "pies" because they are miniature and perfectly portioned. And, in my opinion, they are much easier to make than a full pie!

Yield: 6 to 8 pies

Serving size: 1 pie

DAIRY-FREE, NUT-FREE, SOY-FREE, VEGETARIAN, KID-FRIENDLY

1 pint blueberries
¼ cup honey
1 tablespoon cornstarch
Juice and zest of 1 lemon
1 teaspoon vanilla extract
Pinch salt
1 pie crust dough sheet
Coconut oil spray
1 large egg, beaten
1 teaspoon water

Per serving: Calories: 207; Total fat: 8g; Saturated fat: 1g; Carbohydrate: 33g; Sugar: 19g; Fiber: 2g; Protein: 2g; Sodium: 187mg; Cholesterol: 27mg

1. Preheat the oven to 425°F.

2. Place the blueberries in a small mixing bowl.

3. Add the honey, cornstarch, lemon juice, lemon zest, vanilla, and salt to the bowl and mix well.

4. Roll out the pie crust dough and use the rim of a small drinking glass to cut out four 2½-inch discs.

5. Spray a baking sheet with oil.

6. In a small bowl, combine the egg with the water and beat well.

7. Lay the pie crust circles on the baking sheet and add 1 heaping tablespoon of filling to each circle. Fold the edges of the crust in toward the center, but do not cover the blueberries completely. There should be blueberries showing at the center of each little pie.

8. Brush the edges of the mini pies with the egg wash.

9. Bake in the oven for about 20 minutes, or until the crusts begin to turn golden brown.

Tip: Make the egg wash in a small glass bowl. Save the leftover wash and heat it in the microwave for 1 minute the following morning for a quick breakfast.

LACTATION COOKIES

Prep time: 10 minutes | Cook time: 10 minutes

Lactation cookies are popular among breastfeeding moms. The brewer's yeast in these cookies is thought to help with milk supply, but there are no guarantees on what it will do for your supply. Brewer's yeast is considered an inactive yeast whereas baker's yeast is considered active.

Yield: 12 to 15 cookies

Serving size: 2 cookies

DAIRY-FREE, GLUTEN-FREE, SOY-FREE, GOOD FOR LACTATION, QUICK

1 cup coconut oil
1 cup coconut sugar
2 tablespoons flaxseed meal
4 tablespoons water
2 large eggs
1 teaspoon vanilla extract
2 cups gluten-free oats
4 tablespoons brewer's yeast
1 cup walnut pieces
2 cups chocolate chips
1 cup unsweetened
  coconut flakes
2 cups gluten-free oat flour
1 teaspoon baking soda
1 teaspoon salt
Coconut oil spray

Per serving: Calories: 1351; Total fat: 92g; Saturated fat: 58g; Carbohydrate: 113g; Sugar: 53g; Fiber: 20g; Protein: 23g; Sodium: 662mg; Cholesterol: 55mg

1. Preheat the oven to 350°F.

2. In a large mixing bowl, mix together the coconut oil and the coconut sugar.

3. In a separate small bowl, mix together the flaxseed meal and the water. Add the flaxseed mixture to the coconut sugar mixture and stir to combine.

4. To the large bowl, add the eggs, vanilla, oats, brewer's yeast, walnuts, chocolate chips, and coconut flakes and stir to combine.

5. In a separate large bowl, mix together the oat flour, baking soda, and salt.

6. Add the dry ingredients to the wet ingredients and mix well.

7. Spray a cookie sheet with oil and scoop 1-inch balls of the cookie dough onto the baking sheet, spaced a few inches apart.

8. Bake for about 10 minutes, or until cookies are the desired crispiness.

Tip: If you have a gluten sensitivity, remember to verify that your oats are gluten-free. Also, be sure the chocolate chips are dairy-free if you avoid dairy.

Coconut Macaroons

Prep time: 10 minutes | Cook time: 20 minutes

If you love coconut, try these macaroons. Coconuts are actually fruits, and when they're not accompanied by loads of refined sugar, they provide lots of nutritional benefits, including vitamin B6, iron, magnesium, and zinc.

Yield: 15 macaroons

Serving size:

1 to 2 macaroons

DAIRY-FREE, GLUTEN-FREE, NUT-FREE, SOY-FREE, VEGETARIAN, KID-FRIENDLY, QUICK

4 egg whites
¼ teaspoon salt
¼ cup honey
1 teaspoon vanilla extract
2 cups unsweetened coconut, shredded

Per serving: Calories: 149; Total fat: 10g; Saturated fat: 9g; Carbohydrate: 14g; Sugar: 11g; Fiber: 3g; Protein: 3g; Sodium: 82mg; Cholesterol: 0mg

1. Preheat the oven to 350°F. Line a baking sheet with parchment paper and set aside.

2. In a large bowl, beat the egg whites and salt for about 5 minutes, or until stiff.

3. Fold in the remaining ingredients.

4. Form the dough into tablespoon-size balls and place on the prepared baking sheet.

5. Bake for 10 to 15 minutes, or until the macaroons start to brown.

Tip: It's important to beat the egg whites to just the right stiffness. If you beat them too long or not enough, the mixture may not be thick enough to form into balls.

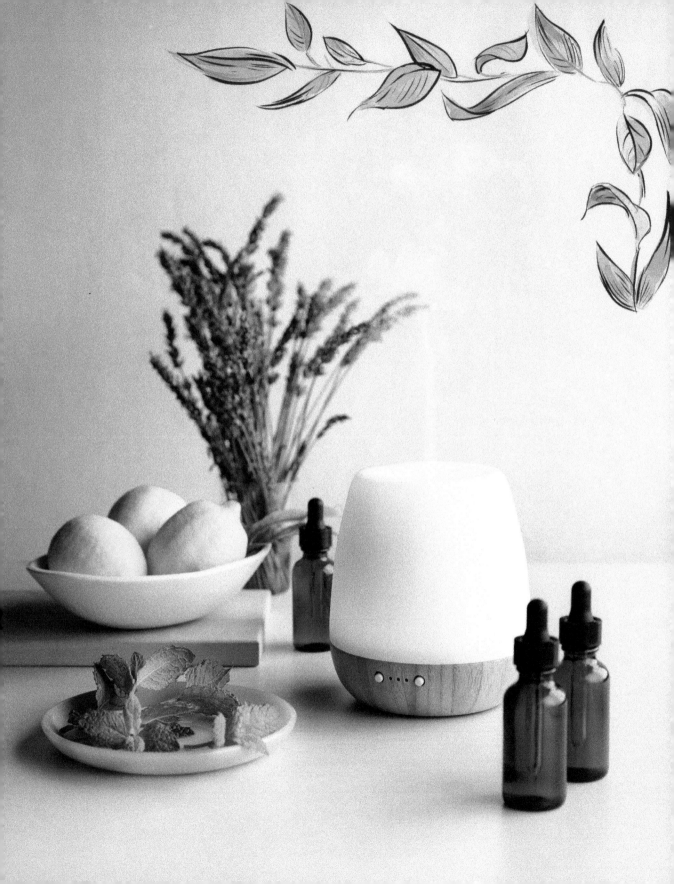

CHAPTER EIGHT

EXTRAS

This chapter includes recipes to help you unwind and find relief from specific pregnancy symptoms.

Nausea-Diffusing Blend

If you are experiencing nausea, one option for relief is to diffuse essential oils. If you don't have a diffuser, look into getting one. They are not expensive and in addition to helping with nausea, they can also improve your relaxation and sleep.

DAIRY-FREE, GLUTEN-FREE,
NUT-FREE, SOY-FREE,
VEGAN, GOOD FOR NAUSEA

4 drops lavender essential oil
2 drops peppermint
  essential oil
1 drop lemon essential oil

1. Fill your diffuser with water to the max line.

2. Add the drops of lavender, peppermint, and lemon one at a time.

3. Set your diffuser next to your bed or your workspace and diffuse for as long as needed. Keep in mind that after three hours you will need to add more drops of essential oil.

Relaxing Face Mask

Prep time: 5 minutes

Who doesn't love a good spa session? I talked about establishing a self-care regimen in chapter 1 (see page 4), and pampering yourself with this face mask is a great way to relax and recharge.

Yield: 1 face mask

DAIRY-FREE, GLUTEN-FREE, NUT-FREE, SOY-FREE, VEGAN, GOOD FOR POSTPARTUM RECOVERY

1 tablespoon coconut oil
1 tablespoon honey
1 teaspoon baking soda

1. Mix the ingredients together in a small bowl.

2. Apply the mask to clean skin and leave it on for about 10 minutes. Rinse it off and feel renewed.

Back Pain Relief Serum

Prep time: 15 minutes | Cook time: 10 minutes

Back pain is a common discomfort during pregnancy for obvious reasons—you are growing a tiny human! Certain stretches, yoga, or meeting with a chiropractor can provide some relief. But you might also want to try this serum.

Yield: 2 cups

DAIRY-FREE, GLUTEN-FREE, NUT-FREE, SOY-FREE, VEGAN

2 cups coconut oil
15 garlic cloves,
   roughly chopped

1. Heat the oil in a small pot over medium-low heat.

2. Add the garlic to the pot and heat until it starts to turn the oil brown.

3. Once fully combined, use a slotted spoon or small strainer to filter the oil and remove the garlic cloves. Let the mixture cool and store it in a glass bottle.

4. Massage the serum on your back before you take a bath or before bed. You can also use it to give yourself a wrist massage.

STRETCH MARK CREAM

Prep time: 8 minutes

There are a lot of products on the market to help prevent or reduce the appearance of stretch marks, but you can easily make your own homemade version with just a handful of all-natural, skin-nourishing ingredients.

Yield: 12 ounces

DAIRY-FREE, GLUTEN-FREE, NUT-FREE, SOY-FREE, GOOD FOR POSTPARTUM RECOVERY, QUICK

½ cup coconut oil
⅓ cup avocado oil
½ cup shea butter
6 drops vitamin E oil
1 scoop marine collagen

1. Combine all the ingredients in a 12-ounce glass jar.

2. Massage a dollop onto your stomach every night, or as much as desired.

Tip: Mark this page for the next time one of your friends is pregnant; this cream makes a great baby shower gift!

Zucchini Bread

Prep time: 10 minutes | Cook time: 50 minutes

This is one of my favorite baked goods to get at a coffee shop, so naturally I had to find a healthier way to make it at home. This recipe is great for when you're craving carbs to combat nausea.

Yield: 8 to 9 servings
Serving size: 1 slice

DAIRY-FREE, SOY-FREE,
VEGETARIAN, GOOD
FOR NAUSEA

3 small or 2 medium to large
    zucchinis, grated
1 large egg
½ cup unsweetened
    applesauce
¾ cup maple syrup
1 teaspoon vanilla extract
1 tablespoon cinnamon
1 teaspoon baking soda
2 teaspoons baking powder
½ teaspoon salt
2 cups whole-wheat flour
⅓ cup walnut pieces, plus
    extra for garnish
Coconut oil spray

1. Preheat the oven to 350°F.
2. Place the zucchini in a medium bowl.
3. In a large mixing bowl, combine the egg, applesauce, maple syrup, and vanilla.
4. To a separate large bowl, add the cinnamon, baking soda, baking powder, and salt. Mix together well.
5. Mix together the dry ingredients with the wet ingredients.
6. Add the zucchini and combine thoroughly. Then fold in the flour slowly, mixing only until it is just combined.
7. Fold in the walnuts.
8. Spray a 9-by-5-inch loaf pan with oil. Scrape the batter into the pan. Sprinkle a few more walnuts on top, if desired.
9. Bake for 50 minutes, or until a toothpick comes out clean.

Per serving: Calories: 256; Total fat: 4g; Saturated fat: 1g; Carbohydrate: 50g; Sugar: 21g; Fiber: 3g; Protein: 6g; Sodium: 327mg; Cholesterol: 23mg

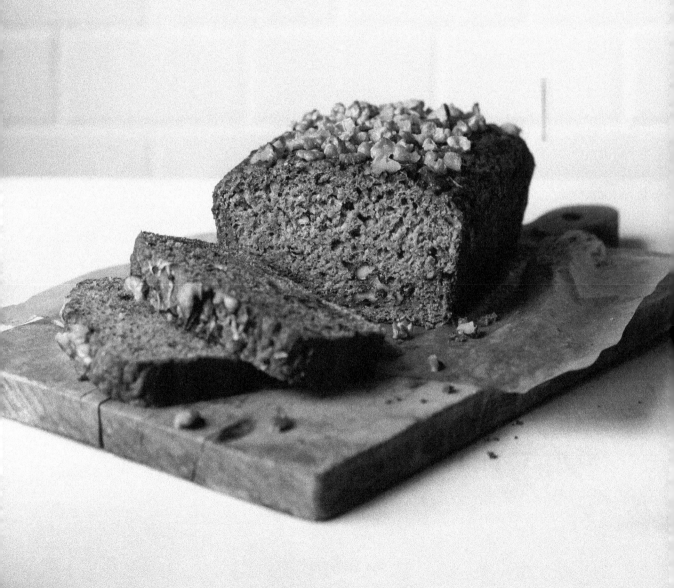

Simple Go-To Salad Dressing

Prep time: 5 minutes

Bottled salad dressings are typically filled with sugar, processed oils, and artificial ingredients. You can make your own dressing in no time, and you likely already have these ingredients in your pantry.

Yield: 1 cup

Serving size:

2 tablespoons

DAIRY-FREE, GLUTEN-FREE, NUT-FREE, SOY-FREE, VEGAN, GESTATIONAL DIABETES–FRIENDLY, QUICK

½ cup extra-virgin olive oil
½ cup balsamic vinegar
1 tablespoon lemon juice
1 tablespoon minced garlic
1 teaspoon Italian seasoning
Pinch salt
Pinch freshly ground
  black pepper

Add all the ingredients to a quart-size mason jar. Cover with a lid and shake to combine.

Per serving: Calories: 115; Total fat: 13g; Saturated fat: 2g; Carbohydrate: 1g; Sugar: 0g; Fiber: 0g; Protein: 0g; Sodium: 21mg; Cholesterol: 0mg

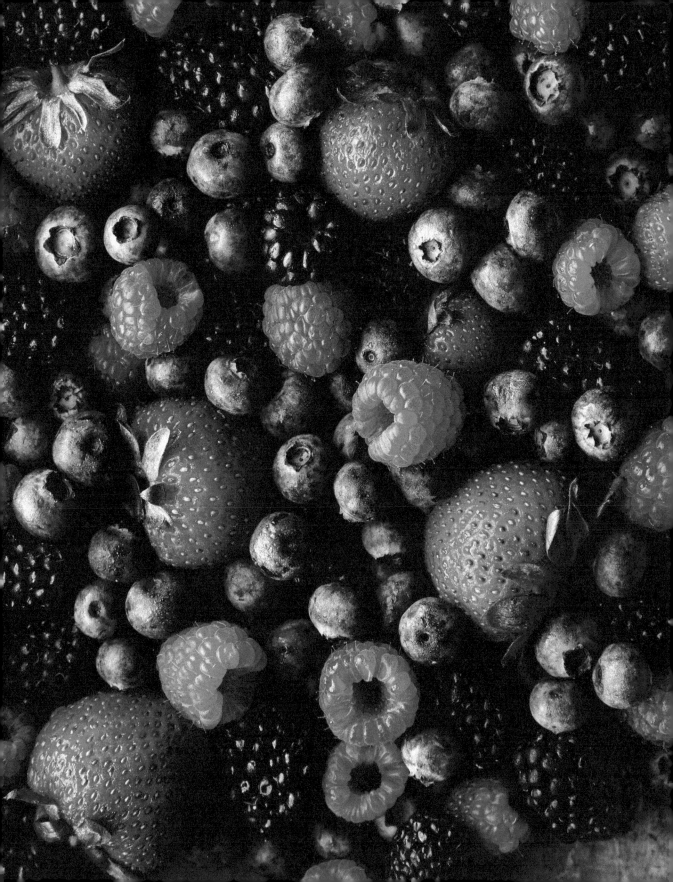

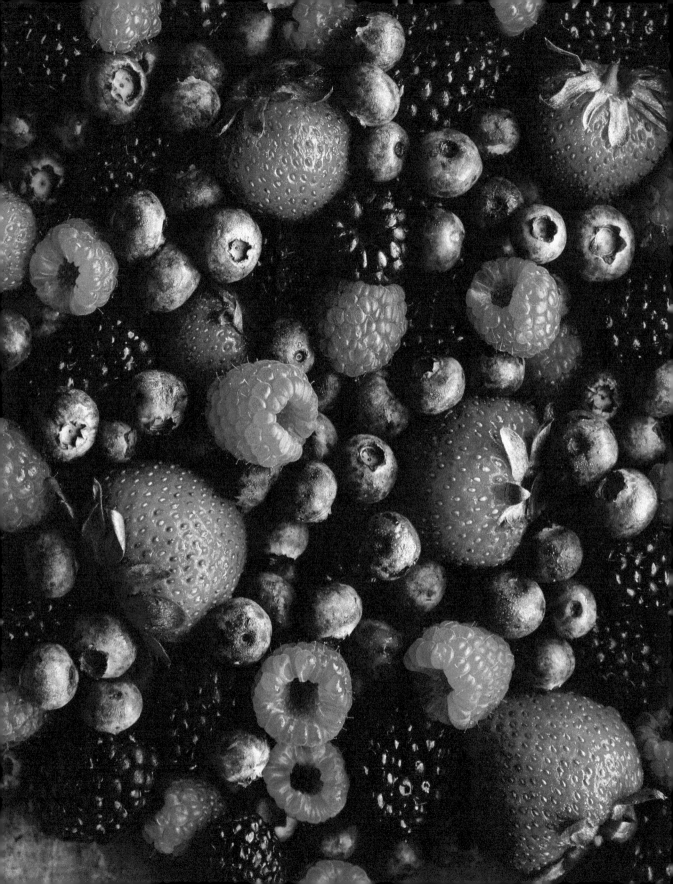

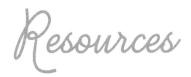
Resources

The American College of Obstetricians and Gynecologists, www.acog.org
This organization of dedicated physicians provides reliable information on all topics relating to women's health and pregnancy.

The Environmental Working Group, www.ewg.org
This group focuses on informing the public about environmental health concerns and is a great resource if you have questions about pesticide use, water quality, or the overall quality of cleaning and beauty supplies. The Environmental Working Group also provides up-to-date news on other popular topics related to helping you live a healthier lifestyle.

***Expect the Best: Your Guide to Healthy Eating Before, During, and After Pregnancy,* 2nd Edition, by Elizabeth M. Ward, MS, RD**
This excellent book provides an overview of nutrition prior to, during, and after pregnancy. It does a good job of providing straightforward recommendations while answering common questions on healthy habits during these pivotal times in life.

March of Dimes, www.marchofdimes.org
This nonprofit agency focuses on advocating for adequate health care for moms and babies. They are at the forefront of research surrounding this population and have resources for consumers and health care professionals.

***Real Food for Gestational Diabetes: An Effective Alternative to the Conventional Nutrition Approach,* by Lily Nichols, RDN, CDE**
This is Lily's first publication and it covers an important and common diagnosis during pregnancy: gestational diabetes. She divulges key nutrition practices and other management tools to ensure you have a healthy pregnancy and baby, even with gestational diabetes.

***Real Food for Pregnancy: The Science and Wisdom of Optimal Prenatal Nutrition,* by Lily Nichols, RDN, CDE**
With more than 900 citations, Lily covers just about every topic related to prenatal nutrition in this groundbreaking book dedicated to changing the way we think about nutrition recommendations during pregnancy and breastfeeding. This book is a truly great tool for any woman who is planning a pregnancy, pregnant, or breastfeeding.

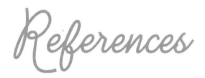

References

Baginski, Leon, Marc Winter, Thomas S. Bailey, Scott Capobianco, et al. "Response to Hydrolysed Collagen Protein Supplementation in a Cohort of Pregnant and Postpartum Women." *Journal of Pregnancy and Child Health* 3, no. 5 (2016). doi:10.4172/2376-127x.1000275.

Chen, Xuyang, Diqi Zhao, Xun Mao, Yinyin Xia, et al. "Maternal Dietary Patterns and Pregnancy Outcome." *Nutrients* 8, no. 6 (June 2016): 351. doi:10.3390/nu8060351.

Dunstan, J. A., K. Simmer, G. Dixon, and S. L. Prescott. "Cognitive Assessment of Children at Age 2½ Years after Maternal Fish Oil Supplementation in Pregnancy: A Randomised Controlled Trial." *Archives of Disease in Childhood: Fetal and Neonatal Edition* 93, no. 1 (January 2008): F45–50. doi:10.1136/adc.2006.099085.

Goletzke, J., A. Buyken, J. Louie, R. Moses, and J. Brand-Miller. "Micronutrient Intake during Pregnancy Is a Function of Carbohydrate Quality," *Journal of Nutrition & Intermediary Metabolism* 1 (2014): 9, https://doi:10.1016/j.jnim.2014.10.181.

Goletzke, J., A. Buyken, R. Moses, and J. Brand-Miller. "Dietary Micronutrient Intake During Pregnancy Is a Function of Carbohydrate Quality," *The American Journal of Clinical Nutrition* 102, no. 3 (September 2015): 626–32. doi:10.3945/ajcn.114.104836.

Jen, Vincent, Nicole S. Erler, Myrte J. Tielemans, Kim V. E. Braun, et al. "Mothers' Intake of Sugar-Containing Beverages During Pregnancy and Body Composition of Their Children During Childhood: The Generation R Study," *The American Journal of Clinical Nutrition* 105, no. 4 (April 2017): 834–41. doi:10.3945/ajcn.116.147934.

March of Dimes. "Morning Sickness," *Pregnancy: Prenatal Care.* Last modified September 2017. Accessed May 1, 2019. https://www.marchofdimes.org/pregnancy/morning-sickness.aspx.

Morrione, Thomas G., and Sam Seifter. "Alteration in the Collagen Content of the Human Uterus During Pregnancy and Post Partum Involution." *Einstein Journal of Biology and Medicine* 24, no. 1 (2016): 32. doi:10.23861/ejbm20082471.

Nichols, Lily. *Real Food for Gestational Diabetes: An Effective Alternative to the Conventional Nutrition Approach.* Kodiak, AL: Lily Nichols, LLC, 2015.

Nichols, Lily. *Real Food for Pregnancy.* Kodiak, AL: Lily Nichols, LLC, 2018.

The Pregnancy Experts at Mayo Clinic. *Mayo Clinic Guide to a Healthy Pregnancy: From Doctors Who Are Parents, Too!* Boston: Da Capo Lifelong Books, 2011.

Ruiz-Gracia, Teresa, Alejandra Duran, Manuel Fuentes, Miguel A. Rubio, et al. "Lifestyle Patterns in Early Pregnancy Linked to Gestational Diabetes Mellitus Diagnoses When Using IADPSG Criteria. The St Carlos Gestational Study." *Clinical Nutrition* 35, no. 3 (June 2016): 699–705. doi:10.1016/j.clnu.2015.04.017.

Sebastiani, Giorgia, Ana Herranz Barbero, Christina Borrás-Novell, Miguel Alsina Casanova, et al. "The Effects of Vegetarian and Vegan Diet during Pregnancy on the Health of Mothers and Offspring." *Nutrients* 11, no. 3 (March 2019): 557. doi:10.3390/nu11030557.

Singh, Meharban. "Essential Fatty Acids, DHA and Human Brain," *The Indian Journal of Pediatrics* 72, no. 3 (March 2005): 239–42. doi:10.1007/bf02859265.

Uriu-Adams, Janet Y., and Carl L. Keen. "Zinc and Reproduction: Effects of Zinc Deficiency on Prenatal and Early Postnatal Development." *Birth Defects Research Part B: Developmental and Reproductive Toxicology* 89, no. 4 (August 2010): 313–25. doi:10.1002/bdrb.20264.

Ward, E. M. *Expect the Best: Your Guide to Healthy Eating Before, During, and After Pregnancy*, 2nd ed. Chicago: The American Dietetic Association, 2017.

Index

A

Almond butter
  Mango Carrot Smoothie, 38
  Sweet Potato Muffins, 41
Almond-Crusted Cod, 81
Amaranth
  Three-Green Ancient Blend, 107
Apples
  Cinnamon Sugar Apples, 135
  Sausage with Apple Sauerkraut
    and Potatoes, 95
  Shredded Brussels Sprouts,
    Apples, and Pecans, 104
Artichoke hearts
  Artichoke, Spinach, and
    White Bean Dip, 120
  Create Your Own Flatbread, 83
  Roasted Veggie Wrap, 82
Arugula
  Citrus Snack Plate, 115
  Scrambled Egg Pita Pocket, 35
  Turkey Arugula Pasta, 93
  Wild Arugula, Spinach,
    and Steak Salad, 55
Asparagus, 16
  Roasted Potatoes, Carrots,
    and Asparagus, 101
Avocados, 16
  Avocado Chicken Salad, 48
  Avocado Chocolate Pudding, 138
  Citrus Snack Plate, 115
  Egg in Tomato Bake, 32
  Kale and Quinoa Salad, 51
  Mahi-Mahi Fish Tacos, 86
  Open-Face Egg Sandwich, 33
  Roasted Veggie Wrap, 82
  Stuffed Avocado
    Salmon Salad, 47
  Taco Jar Salad, 53
  Veggie-Filled Omelet, 39
  Wild Arugula, Spinach,
    and Steak Salad, 55

B

Back pain, 9
Back Pain Relief Serum, 146
Bacon
  Creamy Potato Soup, 65
  Egg, Bacon, and Veggie
    Breakfast Bake, 34
Baked Chicken Legs, 79
Bananas
  Mango Carrot Smoothie, 38
  Sweet Potato Muffins, 41
Beans
  Artichoke, Spinach, and
    White Bean Dip, 120
  Cumin Chicken and
    Black Beans, 80
  Easy Black Bean Burger, 91
  Easy Chicken Chili, 60
  Rustic Italian Salad, 52
  Secret Ingredient Beef Chili, 67
  Simple Veggie Soup, 66
  Taco Jar Salad, 53
Beef
  Beef Stew, 96
  Half Noodle Lasagna, 78
  One-Pot Beef and Broccoli, 75
  Savory Meatballs with
    Egg Noodles, 97
  Secret Ingredient Beef Chili, 67
  Taco Jar Salad, 53
  Wild Arugula, Spinach,
    and Steak Salad, 55
Bell peppers
  Cashew Chicken (or Tempeh)
    Lettuce Wraps, 85
  Chorizo-Potato Hash, 31
  Egg, Bacon, and Veggie
    Breakfast Bake, 34
  Lamb Kabobs, 88
  Open-Face Egg Sandwich, 33
  Pesto Chicken Salad, 49
  Rainbow Fields Salad, 54

  Roasted Veggie Wrap, 82
  Rustic Italian Salad, 52
  Simple Veggie Soup, 66
  Two-Pan Turkey Dinner, 84
Berries, 15
  Berry- and Basil-Infused
    Water, 126
  Berry Parfait, 113
  Blueberry Pecan Pancakes, 28
  Kale and Quinoa Salad, 51
  Mini Blueberry Pies, 139
  Protein-Packed Strawberry
    Smoothie, 37
  Rainbow Fields Salad, 54
  Strawberries and Cream, 133
  Wild Arugula, Spinach,
    and Steak Salad, 55
Blueberry Pecan Pancakes, 28
Bok choy
  Tofu Miso Soup, 68–69
Broccoli, 16
  Broccoli Cream Soup, 62
  Cheesy Mini Quiches, 30
  One-Pot Beef and Broccoli, 75
  Roasted Broccoli with
    Shallots, 102
  Two-Pan Turkey Dinner, 84
Brussels sprouts
  Egg, Bacon, and Veggie
    Breakfast Bake, 34
  Shredded Brussels Sprouts,
    Apples, and Pecans, 104
Butter Lettuce Salad with
  Shrimp, 50

C

Cabbage. *See also* Sauerkraut
  Mahi-Mahi Fish Tacos, 86
  Rainbow Fields Salad, 54
  Simple Coleslaw, 106
Caffeine-Free Vanilla Latte, 128
Caloric needs, 17–18

Carbohydrates, 13–14
Carrots
    Beef Stew, 96
    Carrot Cake for Breakfast, 29
    Cashew Chicken (or Tempeh)
        Lettuce Wraps, 85
    Chicken and Wild Rice Soup, 61
    Mango Carrot Smoothie, 38
    Rainbow Fields Salad, 54
    Roasted Potatoes, Carrots,
        and Asparagus, 101
    Rustic Italian Salad, 52
    Simple Veggie Soup, 66
    Two-Pan Turkey Dinner, 84
    Warm Lentil and Kale Soup, 59
Cashew Chicken (or Tempeh)
    Lettuce Wraps, 85
Cauliflower
    Cauliflower Mash, 108
    Protein-Packed
        Strawberry Smoothie, 37
Cheddar cheese
    Broccoli Cream Soup, 62
    Cheesy Mini Quiches, 30
    Classic Tomato Soup and
        Grilled Cheese, 57–58
    Creamy Potato Soup, 65
Cheese. See specific
Cheesy Mini Quiches, 30
Chia seeds, 15
    Berry Parfait, 113
    Kale and Quinoa Salad, 51
    Kiwi, Cucumber,
        Kale Smoothie, 40
    Peanut Butter Energy Bites, 112
    Seedy Chocolate Bark, 136
Chicken
    Avocado Chicken Salad, 48
    Baked Chicken Legs, 79
    Cashew Chicken (or Tempeh)
        Lettuce Wraps, 85
    Chicken and Wild Rice Soup, 61
    Create Your Own Flatbread, 83
    Cumin Chicken and
        Black Beans, 80
    Easy Chicken Chili, 60
    One-Pan Chicken and
        Chickpea Bake, 72

Pesto Chicken Salad, 49
    Rainbow Chard–Stuffed
        Chicken Breasts, 76
    Rustic Italian Salad, 52
Chickpeas
    Fresh Veggie Couscous, 109
    Kale and Quinoa Salad, 51
    One-Pan Chicken and
        Chickpea Bake, 72
    Roasted Chickpeas, 114
    Roasted Veggie Wrap, 82
    Turmeric Hummus, 111
Chiles, green
    Easy Chicken Chili, 60
Chocolate
    Avocado Chocolate
        Pudding, 138
    Dark Chocolate–Covered
        Raisins, 134
    Lactation Cookies, 140
    Peanut Butter Energy Bites, 112
    Seedy Chocolate Bark, 136
Chorizo-Potato Hash, 31
Cinnamon Sugar Apples, 135
Citrus Snack Plate, 115
Classic Deviled Eggs, 121
Classic Tomato Soup and
    Grilled Cheese, 57–58
Coconut
    Berry Parfait, 113
    Carrot Cake for Breakfast, 29
    Coconut Macaroons, 141
    Lactation Cookies, 140
    Peanut Butter Energy Bites, 112
Cod, Almond-Crusted, 81
Constipation, 8
Corn
    Easy Chicken Chili, 60
    Edamame Frittata, 42
    Taco Jar Salad, 53
Couscous, Fresh Veggie, 109
Crave-Worthy Egg Salad, 46
Cream cheese
    Artichoke, Spinach, and
        White Bean Dip, 120
    Chicken and Wild Rice Soup, 61
    Spinach Parmesan
        Spaghetti Squash, 89

Creamy Potato Soup, 65
Create Your Own Flatbread, 83
Crustless Spinach Quiche, 43
Cucumbers
    Fresh Veggie Couscous, 109
    Kale and Quinoa Salad, 51
    Kiwi, Cucumber,
        Kale Smoothie, 40
    Knockout Nausea Water, 125
Cumin Chicken and
    Black Beans, 80

D

Dairy-free diets, 20
Dairy-free recipes
    Almond-Crusted Cod, 81
    Avocado Chicken Salad, 48
    Back Pain Relief Serum, 146
    Baked Chicken Legs, 79
    Beef Stew, 96
    Berry- and Basil-Infused
        Water, 126
    Caffeine-Free Vanilla Latte, 128
    Carrot Cake for Breakfast, 29
    Cashew Chicken (or Tempeh)
        Lettuce Wraps, 85
    Chorizo-Potato Hash, 31
    Citrus Snack Plate, 115
    Coconut Macaroons, 141
    Crave-Worthy Egg Salad, 46
    Delicata Squash Soup, 63–64
    Easy Black Bean Burger, 91
    Egg in Tomato Bake, 32
    Electrolyte Balance, 127
    Fresh Veggie Couscous, 109
    Half Noodle Lasagna, 78
    Home-Baked Kale Chips, 119
    Kale and Quinoa Salad, 51
    Kiwi, Cucumber, Kale
        Smoothie, 40
    Knockout Nausea Water, 125
    Lactation Cookies, 140
    Lactation Tea Blend, 129
    Lamb Kabobs, 88
    Lemony Garlic Shrimp, 73
    Mango Carrot Smoothie, 38
    Mediterranean Roasted
        Salmon, 92

Dairy-free recipes *(continued)*
Mini Blueberry Pies, 139
Nausea-Diffusing Blend, 144
One-Pan Chicken and
Chickpea Bake, 72
One-Pot Beef and Broccoli, 75
Pineapple Mojito Mocktail, 131
Rainbow Fields Salad, 54
Relaxing Face Mask, 145
Roasted Broccoli
with Shallots, 102
Roasted Chickpeas, 114
Roasted Potatoes, Carrots,
and Asparagus, 101
Roasted Veggie Wrap, 82
Secret Ingredient Beef Chili, 67
Shredded Brussels Sprouts,
Apples, and Pecans, 104
Simple Go-To Salad
Dressing, 150
Simple Veggie Soup, 66
Slow-Cooked Pulled Pork, 77
Stretch Mark Cream, 147
Sugar-Free Freshly Squeezed
Lemonade, 130
Sweet Potato Fries, 103
Sweet Potato Muffins, 41
Three-Grain Ancient Blend, 107
Tofu Miso Soup, 68–69
Tofu Stir-Fry, 94
Turkey Arugula Pasta, 93
Turmeric Hummus, 111
Two-Pan Turkey Dinner, 84
Veggie-Filled Omelet, 39
Warm Lentil and Kale Soup, 59
Zucchini Bread, 148
Dark Chocolate–Covered
Raisins, 134
Delicata Squash Soup, 63–64

E

Easy Black Bean Burger, 91
Easy Chicken Chili, 60
"Eating for two," 12
Edamame Frittata, 42

Eggs, 15
Blueberry Pecan Pancakes, 28
Cheesy Mini Quiches, 30
Chorizo-Potato Hash, 31
Classic Deviled Eggs, 121
Coconut Macaroons, 141
Crave-Worthy Egg Salad, 46
Crustless Spinach Quiche, 43
Edamame Frittata, 42
Egg, Bacon, and Veggie
Breakfast Bake, 34
Egg in Tomato Bake, 32
Lactation Cookies, 140
Open-Face Egg Sandwich, 33
Rainbow Fields Salad, 54
Scrambled Egg Pita
Pocket, 35
Tofu Stir-Fry, 94
Veggie-Filled Omelet, 39
Electrolyte Balance, 127
Equipment, 24–25
Essential oils
Nausea-Diffusing Blend, 144

F

Fats, 13–14
Fennel
Mediterranean Roasted
Salmon, 92
Feta cheese
Lentil and Quinoa
"Meat"balls, 74
Scrambled Egg Pita Pocket, 35
Fish
Almond-Crusted Cod, 81
Mahi-Mahi Fish Tacos, 86
Mediterranean Roasted
Salmon, 92
Pan-Seared Rainbow Trout, 90
salmon, 15
Stuffed Avocado
Salmon Salad, 47
Food safety, 25
Fresh Veggie Couscous, 109

G

Gestational diabetes
mellitus (GDM), 18
Gluten-free diets, 20
Gluten-free recipes
Almond-Crusted Cod, 81
Artichoke, Spinach, and
White Bean Dip, 120
Avocado Chicken Salad, 48
Avocado Chocolate Pudding, 138
Back Pain Relief Serum, 146
Baked Chicken Legs, 79
Berry- and Basil-Infused
Water, 126
Berry Parfait, 113
Blueberry Pecan Pancakes, 28
Broccoli Cream Soup, 62
Butter Lettuce Salad
with Shrimp, 50
Caffeine-Free Vanilla Latte, 128
Cashew Chicken (or Tempeh)
Lettuce Wraps, 85
Cauliflower Mash, 108
Chicken and Wild Rice Soup, 61
Chorizo-Potato Hash, 31
Cinnamon Sugar Apples, 135
Citrus Snack Plate, 115
Classic Deviled Eggs, 121
Creamy Potato Soup, 65
Crustless Spinach Quiche, 43
Cumin Chicken and
Black Beans, 80
Dark Chocolate–Covered
Raisins, 134
Delicata Squash Soup, 63–64
Easy Black Bean Burger, 91
Easy Chicken Chili, 60
Egg, Bacon, and Veggie
Breakfast Bake, 34
Egg in Tomato Bake, 32
Electrolyte Balance, 127
Home-Baked Kale Chips, 119
Kale and Quinoa Salad, 51
Kiwi, Cucumber, Kale
Smoothie, 40

Knockout Nausea Water, 125
Lactation Cookies, 140
Lactation Tea Blend, 129
Lamb Kabobs, 88
Lemony Garlic Shrimp, 73
Lentil and Quinoa
    "Meat"balls, 74
Mahi-Mahi Fish Tacos, 86
Mango Carrot Smoothie, 38
Mediterranean
    Roasted Salmon, 92
Mozzarella Bites, 116
Nausea-Diffusing Blend, 144
One-Pan Chicken and
    Chickpea Bake, 72
One-Pot Beef and Broccoli, 75
Pan-Seared Rainbow Trout, 90
Parmesan Green Beans
    and Mushrooms, 105
Peanut Butter Energy Bites, 112
Pesto Chicken Salad, 49
Pineapple Mojito Mocktail, 131
Protein-Packed Strawberry
    Smoothie, 37
Rainbow Chard–Stuffed
    Chicken Breasts, 76
Rainbow Fields Salad, 54
Relaxing Face Mask, 145
Roasted Broccoli
    with Shallots, 102
Roasted Chickpeas, 114
Roasted Potatoes, Carrots,
    and Asparagus, 101
Roasted Veggie Wrap, 82
Rustic Italian Salad, 52
Sausage with Apple Sauerkraut
    and Potatoes, 95
Scrambled Egg Pita Pocket, 35
Seedy Chocolate Bark, 136
Shredded Brussels Sprouts,
    Apples, and Pecans, 104
Simple Coleslaw, 106
Simple Go-To Salad
    Dressing, 150
Simple Veggie Soup, 66

Slow-Cooked Pulled Pork, 77
Spinach Parmesan
    Spaghetti Squash, 89
Strawberries and Cream, 133
Stretch Mark Cream, 147
Stuffed Avocado Salmon
    Salad, 47
Sugar-Free Freshly Squeezed
    Lemonade, 130
Sweet Potato Fries, 103
Sweet Potato Muffins, 41
Taco Jar Salad, 53
Three-Grain Ancient
    Blend, 107
Traditional Caprese Salad, 117
Turmeric Hummus, 111
Two-Pan Turkey Dinner, 84
Veggie-Filled Omelet, 39
Warm Lentil and Kale Soup, 59
Wild Arugula, Spinach,
    and Steak Salad, 55
Goat cheese
    Edamame Frittata, 42
    Shredded Brussels Sprouts,
        Apples, and Pecans, 104
Gorgonzola cheese
    Wild Arugula, Spinach,
        and Steak Salad, 55
Grapefruits
    Citrus Snack Plate, 115
Greek yogurt, 16
    Berry Parfait, 113
    Protein-Packed Strawberry
        Smoothie, 37
    Simple Coleslaw, 106
Green beans and Mushrooms,
    Parmesan, 105
Greens. *See also specific*
    Rainbow Fields Salad, 54

H

Half Noodle Lasagna, 78
Health-care providers, 6
Heartburn, 8
Home-Baked Kale Chips, 119

I

Iron, 8

K

Kale, 16
    Home-Baked Kale Chips, 119
    Kale and Quinoa Salad, 51
    Kiwi, Cucumber, Kale
        Smoothie, 40
    Veggie-Filled Omelet, 39
    Warm Lentil and Kale Soup, 59
Keto diets, 20
Kid-friendly recipes
    Almond-Crusted Cod, 81
    Avocado Chocolate Pudding, 138
    Baked Chicken Legs, 79
    Beef Stew, 96
    Blueberry Pecan Pancakes, 28
    Broccoli Cream Soup, 62
    Carrot Cake for Breakfast, 29
    Cashew Chicken (or Tempeh)
        Lettuce Wraps, 85
    Cheesy Mini Quiches, 30
    Classic Deviled Eggs, 121
    Classic Tomato Soup and
        Grilled Cheese, 57–58
    Coconut Macaroons, 141
    Creamy Potato Soup, 65
    Create Your Own Flatbread, 83
    Cumin Chicken and
        Black Beans, 80
    Dark Chocolate–Covered
        Raisins, 134
    Egg, Bacon, and Veggie
        Breakfast Bake, 34
    Half Noodle Lasagna, 78
    Lamb Kabobs, 88
    Mango Carrot Smoothie, 38
    Mini Blueberry Pies, 139
    Mozzarella Bites, 116
    Peanut Butter Energy Bites, 112
    Pesto Chicken Salad, 49
    Protein-Packed Strawberry
        Smoothie, 37

Savory Meatballs with
Egg Noodles, 97
Scrambled Egg Pita Pocket, 35
Secret Ingredient Beef Chili, 67
Simple Veggie Soup, 66
Slow-Cooked Pulled Pork, 77
Sugar-Free Freshly
Squeezed Lemonade, 130
Sweet Potato Fries, 103
Sweet Potato Muffins, 41
Taco Jar Salad, 53
Turkey Arugula Pasta, 93
Kiwi, Cucumber, Kale
Smoothie, 40
Knockout Nausea Water, 125

L

Lactation Cookies, 140
Lactation Tea Blend, 129
Lamb Kabobs, 88
Leg cramps, 9
Lemony Garlic Shrimp, 73
Lentils, 16
Lentil and Quinoa
"Meat"balls, 74
Warm Lentil and Kale Soup, 59
Lettuce
Butter Lettuce Salad
with Shrimp, 50
Cashew Chicken (or Tempeh)
Lettuce Wraps, 85
Rustic Italian Salad, 52
Taco Jar Salad, 53

M

Mahi-Mahi Fish Tacos, 86
Mango Carrot Smoothie, 38
Mediterranean
Roasted Salmon, 92
Mexican cheese blend
Cumin Chicken and
Black Beans, 80
Taco Jar Salad, 53
Millet
Three-Grain Ancient Blend, 107
Mini Blueberry Pies, 139

Miso paste
Tofu Miso Soup, 68–69
Morning sickness, 2, 7, 27
Mozzarella cheese
Create Your Own Flatbread, 83
Crustless Spinach Quiche, 43
Half Noodle Lasagna, 78
Mozzarella Bites, 116
Traditional Caprese Salad, 117
Multiples, 18
Mushrooms
Chicken and Wild Rice Soup, 61
Lamb Kabobs, 88
Parmesan Green Beans
and Mushrooms, 105
Roasted Veggie Wrap, 82
Veggie-Filled Omelet, 39
Warm Lentil and Kale Soup, 59

N

Nausea, 2, 7
Nausea-Diffusing Blend, 144
Noodles
Half Noodle Lasagna, 78
Savory Meatballs with
Egg Noodles, 97
Tofu Miso Soup, 68–69
Nut-free recipes
Artichoke, Spinach, and
White Bean Dip, 120
Avocado Chicken Salad, 48
Avocado Chocolate Pudding, 138
Back Pain Relief Serum, 146
Baked Chicken Legs, 79
Beef Stew, 96
Berry- and Basil-Infused
Water, 126
Broccoli Cream Soup, 62
Cauliflower Mash, 108
Cheesy Mini Quiches, 30
Chicken and Wild Rice Soup, 61
Chorizo-Potato Hash, 31
Citrus Snack Plate, 115
Classic Deviled Eggs, 121
Classic Tomato Soup and
Grilled Cheese, 57–58

Coconut Macaroons, 141
Crave-Worthy Egg Salad, 46
Creamy Potato Soup, 65
Create Your Own Flatbread, 83
Crustless Spinach Quiche, 43
Cumin Chicken and
Black Beans, 80
Dark Chocolate–Covered
Raisins, 134
Delicata Squash Soup, 63–64
Easy Black Bean Burger, 91
Easy Chicken Chili, 60
Edamame Frittata, 42
Egg, Bacon, and Veggie
Breakfast Bake, 34
Electrolyte Balance, 127
Fresh Veggie Couscous, 109
Half Noodle Lasagna, 78
Home-Baked Kale Chips, 119
Knockout Nausea Water, 125
Lamb Kabobs, 88
Lemony Garlic Shrimp, 73
Mahi-Mahi Fish Tacos, 86
Mediterranean Roasted
Salmon, 92
Mini Blueberry Pies, 139
Nausea-Diffusing Blend, 144
One-Pan Chicken and
Chickpea Bake, 72
One-Pot Beef and Broccoli, 75
Open-Face Egg Sandwich, 33
Pan-Seared Rainbow Trout, 90
Parmesan Green Beans
and Mushrooms, 105
Pineapple Mojito Mocktail, 131
Protein-Packed Strawberry
Smoothie, 37
Rainbow Chard–Stuffed
Chicken Breasts, 76
Relaxing Face Mask, 145
Roasted Broccoli with
Shallots, 102
Roasted Chickpeas, 114
Roasted Potatoes, Carrots,
and Asparagus, 101
Roasted Veggie Wrap, 82

Rustic Italian Salad, 52
Sausage with Apple Sauerkraut
　　and Potatoes, 95
Savory Meatballs with
　　Egg Noodles, 97
Scrambled Egg Pita Pocket, 35
Secret Ingredient Beef
　　Chili, 67
Seedy Chocolate Bark, 136
Simple Coleslaw, 106
Simple Go-To Salad
　　Dressing, 150
Simple Veggie Soup, 66
Slow-Cooked Pulled Pork, 77
Spinach Parmesan
　　Spaghetti Squash, 89
Strawberries and Cream, 133
Stretch Mark Cream, 147
Stuffed Avocado Salmon
　　Salad, 47
Sugar-Free Freshly Squeezed
　　Lemonade, 130
Sweet Potato Fries, 103
Three-Grain Ancient Blend, 107
Tofu Miso Soup, 68–69
Tofu Stir-Fry, 94
Traditional Caprese Salad, 117
Turkey Arugula Pasta, 93
Turmeric Hummus, 111
Two-Pan Turkey Dinner, 84
Veggie-Filled Omelet, 39
Warm Lentil and Kale Soup, 59
Nutrition, 12–18
Nuts
　　Almond-Crusted Cod, 81
　　Berry Parfait, 113
　　Blueberry Pecan Pancakes, 28
　　Butter Lettuce Salad
　　　　with Shrimp, 50
　　Carrot Cake for Breakfast, 29
　　Cashew Chicken (or Tempeh)
　　　　Lettuce Wraps, 85
　　Cinnamon Sugar Apples, 135
　　Kale and Quinoa Salad, 51
　　Lactation Cookies, 140
　　Rainbow Fields Salad, 54

Shredded Brussels Sprouts,
　　Apples, and Pecans, 104
Wild Arugula, Spinach,
　　and Steak Salad, 55
Zucchini Bread, 148

O
Oats
　　Carrot Cake for Breakfast, 29
　　Easy Black Bean Burger, 91
　　Lactation Cookies, 140
　　Peanut Butter Energy Bites, 112
　　Sweet Potato Muffins, 41
One-Pan Chicken and Chickpea
　　Bake, 72
One-Pot Beef and Broccoli, 75
Open-Face Egg Sandwich, 33
Oranges
　　Citrus Snack Plate, 115

P
Paleo diets, 20
Pan-Seared Rainbow Trout, 90
Pantry staples, 24
Parmesan cheese
　　Artichoke, Spinach, and
　　　　White Bean Dip, 120
　　Create Your Own Flatbread, 83
　　Parmesan Green Beans
　　　　and Mushrooms, 105
　　Pesto Chicken Salad, 49
　　Rainbow Chard–Stuffed
　　　　Chicken Breasts, 76
　　Rustic Italian Salad, 52
　　Spinach Parmesan
　　　　Spaghetti Squash, 89
Pasta, Turkey Arugula, 93
Peanut Butter Energy
　　Bites, 112
Peas
　　Beef Stew, 96
Pescatarian diets, 20
Pesto Chicken Salad, 49
Pineapple Mojito Mocktail, 131
Pork. See also Bacon; Sausage
　　Slow-Cooked Pulled Pork, 77

Potatoes. See also Sweet potatoes
　　Beef Stew, 96
　　Chorizo-Potato Hash, 31
　　Creamy Potato Soup, 65
　　Roasted Potatoes, Carrots,
　　　　and Asparagus, 101
　　Sausage with Apple Sauerkraut
　　　　and Potatoes, 95
Pregnancy
　　first trimester, 7
　　health during, 2
　　nutrition during, 12–18
　　second trimester, 8
　　third trimester, 9
　　what to expect, 6
Processed foods, 13
Protein, 13–14
Protein-Packed Strawberry
　　Smoothie, 37
Pumpkin purée
　　Carrot Cake for Breakfast, 29

Q
Quick recipes
　　Artichoke, Spinach, and
　　　　White Bean Dip, 120
　　Berry- and Basil-Infused
　　　　Water, 126
　　Berry Parfait, 113
　　Butter Lettuce Salad
　　　　with Shrimp, 50
　　Caffeine-Free Vanilla Latte, 128
　　Chorizo-Potato Hash, 31
　　Citrus Snack Plate, 115
　　Classic Deviled Eggs, 121
　　Coconut Macaroons, 141
　　Crave-Worthy Egg Salad, 46
　　Create Your Own Flatbread, 83
　　Crustless Spinach Quiche, 43
　　Dark Chocolate–Covered
　　　　Raisins, 134
　　Easy Black Bean Burger, 91
　　Easy Chicken Chili, 60
　　Edamame Frittata, 42
　　Home-Baked Kale Chips, 119
　　Kale and Quinoa Salad, 51

Quick recipes *(continued)*

Kiwi, Cucumber, Kale
Smoothie, 40

Lactation Cookies, 140

Mango Carrot Smoothie, 38

Mozzarella Bites, 116

Open-Face Egg Sandwich, 33

Pan-Seared Rainbow Trout, 90

Parmesan Green Beans
and Mushrooms, 105

Pesto Chicken Salad, 49

Pineapple Mojito Mocktail, 131

Protein-Packed Strawberry
Smoothie, 37

Roasted Broccoli with
Shallots, 102

Roasted Veggie Wrap, 82

Rustic Italian Salad, 52

Scrambled Egg Pita Pocket, 35

Seedy Chocolate Bark, 136

Shredded Brussels Sprouts,
Apples, and Pecans, 104

Simple Coleslaw, 106

Simple Go-To Salad
Dressing, 150

Strawberries and Cream, 133

Stretch Mark Cream, 147

Stuffed Avocado Salmon
Salad, 47

Sugar-Free Freshly Squeezed
Lemonade, 130

Traditional Caprese Salad, 117

Turmeric Hummus, 111

Two-Pan Turkey Dinner, 84

Veggie-Filled Omelet, 39

Quinoa

Kale and Quinoa Salad, 51

Lentil and Quinoa
"Meat"balls, 74

R

Radishes

Rainbow Fields Salad, 54

Rainbow Chard–Stuffed Chicken
Breasts, 76

Rainbow Fields Salad, 54

Raisins

Carrot Cake for Breakfast, 29

Dark Chocolate–Covered
Raisins, 134

Recipes, about, 22–23

Relaxing Face Mask, 145

Rice

Chicken and Wild Rice Soup, 61

Tofu Stir-Fry, 94

Ricotta cheese

Create Your Own Flatbread, 83

Half Noodle Lasagna, 78

Roasted Broccoli with
Shallots, 102

Roasted Chickpeas, 114

Roasted Potatoes, Carrots, and
Asparagus, 101

Roasted Veggie Wrap, 82

Rustic Italian Salad, 52

S

Salmon, 15

Mediterranean Roasted
Salmon, 92

Stuffed Avocado Salmon
Salad, 47

Sauerkraut

Sausage with Apple Sauerkraut
and Potatoes, 95

Sausage

Chorizo-Potato Hash, 31

Sausage with Apple Sauerkraut
and Potatoes, 95

Savory Meatballs with Egg
Noodles, 97

Scrambled Egg Pita Pocket, 35

Secret Ingredient Beef Chili, 67

Seedy Chocolate Bark, 136

Self-care, 4–5

Relaxing Face Mask, 145

Shredded Brussels Sprouts,
Apples, and Pecans, 104

Shrimp

Butter Lettuce Salad
with Shrimp, 50

Lemony Garlic Shrimp, 73

Simple Coleslaw, 106

Simple Go-To Salad Dressing, 150

Simple Veggie Soup, 66

Slow-Cooked Pulled Pork, 77

Soy-free recipes

Artichoke, Spinach, and
White Bean Dip, 120

Avocado Chicken Salad, 48

Avocado Chocolate
Pudding, 138

Back Pain Relief Serum, 146

Baked Chicken Legs, 79

Beef Stew, 96

Berry- and Basil-Infused
Water, 126

Berry Parfait, 113

Blueberry Pecan Pancakes, 28

Broccoli Cream Soup, 62

Butter Lettuce Salad
with Shrimp, 50

Caffeine-Free Vanilla Latte, 128

Cauliflower Mash, 108

Cheesy Mini Quiches, 30

Chicken and Wild Rice Soup, 61

Chorizo-Potato Hash, 31

Cinnamon Sugar Apples, 135

Citrus Snack Plate, 115

Classic Deviled Eggs, 121

Classic Tomato Soup and
Grilled Cheese, 57–58

Coconut Macaroons, 141

Creamy Potato Soup, 65

Create Your Own Flatbread, 83

Crustless Spinach Quiche, 43

Cumin Chicken and
Black Beans, 80

Dark Chocolate–Covered
Raisins, 134

Delicata Squash Soup, 63–64

Easy Black Bean Burger, 91

Easy Chicken Chili, 60

Egg, Bacon, and Veggie
Breakfast Bake, 34

Electrolyte Balance, 127

Fresh Veggie Couscous, 109

Half Noodle Lasagna, 78

Home-Baked Kale Chips, 119
Kale and Quinoa Salad, 51
Kiwi, Cucumber, Kale
    Smoothie, 40
Lactation Cookies, 140
Lactation Tea Blend, 129
Lamb Kabobs, 88
Lemony Garlic Shrimp, 73
Lentil and Quinoa
    "Meat"balls, 74
Mahi-Mahi Fish Tacos, 86
Mango Carrot Smoothie, 38
Mediterranean Roasted
    Salmon, 92
Mini Blueberry Pies, 139
Mozzarella Bites, 116
Nausea-Diffusing Blend, 144
One-Pan Chicken and
    Chickpea Bake, 72
Open-Face Egg Sandwich, 33
Pan-Seared Rainbow Trout, 90
Parmesan Green Beans
    and Mushrooms, 105
Peanut Butter Energy Bites, 112
Pesto Chicken Salad, 49
Pineapple Mojito Mocktail, 131
Protein-Packed Strawberry
    Smoothie, 37
Rainbow Fields Salad, 54
Relaxing Face Mask, 145
Roasted Broccoli with
    Shallots, 102
Roasted Chickpeas, 114
Roasted Potatoes, Carrots,
    and Asparagus, 101
Roasted Veggie Wrap, 82
Rustic Italian Salad, 52
Sausage with Apple Sauerkraut
    and Potatoes, 95
Savory Meatballs with
    Egg Noodles, 97
Scrambled Egg Pita Pocket, 35
Secret Ingredient Beef Chili, 67
Seedy Chocolate Bark, 136
Shredded Brussels Sprouts,
    Apples, and Pecans, 104

Simple Coleslaw, 106
Simple Go-To Salad
    Dressing, 150
Simple Veggie Soup, 66
Slow-Cooked Pulled Pork, 77
Spinach Parmesan
    Spaghetti Squash, 89
Strawberries and Cream, 133
Stretch Mark Cream, 147
Stuffed Avocado Salmon
    Salad, 47
Sugar-Free Freshly Squeezed
    Lemonade, 130
Sweet Potato Fries, 103
Sweet Potato Muffins, 41
Taco Jar Salad, 53
Three-Grain Ancient
    Blend, 107
Traditional Caprese Salad, 117
Turkey Arugula Pasta, 93
Turmeric Hummus, 111
Two-Pan Turkey Dinner, 84
Veggie-Filled Omelet, 39
Warm Lentil and Kale Soup, 59
Wild Arugula, Spinach,
    and Steak Salad, 55
Zucchini Bread, 148
Spinach
    Artichoke, Spinach, and
        White Bean Dip, 120
    Create Your Own Flatbread, 83
    Crustless Spinach Quiche, 43
    Mango Carrot Smoothie, 38
    Open-Face Egg Sandwich, 33
    Spinach Parmesan
        Spaghetti Squash, 89
    Wild Arugula, Spinach,
        and Steak Salad, 55
Squash. See also Zucchini
    Delicata Squash Soup, 63–64
    Simple Veggie Soup, 66
    Spinach Parmesan
        Spaghetti Squash, 89
Strawberries and Cream, 133
Stretch Mark Cream, 147
Stuffed Avocado Salmon Salad, 47

Sugar-Free Freshly Squeezed
    Lemonade, 130
Supplements, 12
Sweet potatoes
    Simple Veggie Soup, 66
    Sweet Potato Fries, 103
    Sweet Potato Muffins, 41
Swelling, 9

T
Taco Jar Salad, 53
Teff
    Rainbow Fields Salad, 54
    Three-Grain Ancient Blend, 107
    Three-Green Ancient Blend, 107
Tofu Miso Soup, 68–69
Tofu Stir-Fry, 94
Tomatoes
    Classic Tomato Soup and
        Grilled Cheese, 57–58
    Create Your Own Flatbread, 83
    Egg in Tomato Bake, 32
    Fresh Veggie Couscous, 109
    Mediterranean Roasted
        Salmon, 92
    One-Pan Chicken and
        Chickpea Bake, 72
    Rustic Italian Salad, 52
    Scrambled Egg Pita Pocket, 35
    Secret Ingredient Beef Chili, 67
    Taco Jar Salad, 53
    Traditional Caprese Salad, 117
Tomatoes, sun-dried
    Turkey Arugula Pasta, 93
Traditional Caprese Salad, 117
Trout, Pan-Seared Rainbow, 90
Turkey
    Turkey Arugula Pasta, 93
    Two-Pan Turkey Dinner, 84
Turmeric Hummus, 111
Two-Pan Turkey Dinner, 84

V
Vegan diets, 19
Vegan recipes
    Back Pain Relief Serum, 146

Vegan recipes *(continued)*
 Berry- and Basil-Infused
  Water, 126
 Citrus Snack Plate, 115
 Delicata Squash Soup, 63–64
 Easy Black Bean Burger, 91
 Electrolyte Balance, 127
 Fresh Veggie Couscous, 109
 Home-Baked Kale Chips, 119
 Kale and Quinoa Salad, 51
 Kiwi, Cucumber, Kale
  Smoothie, 40
 Knockout Nausea Water, 125
 Lactation Tea Blend, 129
 Mango Carrot Smoothie, 38
 Nausea-Diffusing Blend, 144
 Relaxing Face Mask, 145
 Roasted Broccoli with
  Shallots, 102
 Roasted Chickpeas, 114
 Roasted Potatoes, Carrots,
  and Asparagus, 101
 Roasted Veggie Wrap, 82
 Simple Go-To Salad
  Dressing, 150
 Simple Veggie Soup, 66
 Sugar-Free Freshly Squeezed
  Lemonade, 130
 Sweet Potato Fries, 103
 Sweet Potato Muffins, 41
 Three-Grain Ancient Blend, 107
 Turmeric Hummus, 111

Vegetables. *See also specific*
 Tofu Stir-Fry, 94
Vegetarian diets, 19
Vegetarian recipes. *See also*
 Vegan recipes
 Artichoke, Spinach, and
  White Bean Dip, 120
 Avocado Chocolate
  Pudding, 138
 Berry Parfait, 113
 Blueberry Pecan Pancakes, 28
 Broccoli Cream Soup, 62
 Cauliflower Mash, 108
 Cheesy Mini Quiches, 30
 Cinnamon Sugar Apples, 135
 Classic Deviled Eggs, 121
 Classic Tomato Soup and
  Grilled Cheese, 57–58
 Coconut Macaroons, 141
 Crave-Worthy Egg Salad, 46
 Crustless Spinach Quiche, 43
 Edamame Frittata, 42
 Egg in Tomato Bake, 32
 Lentil and Quinoa
  "Meat"balls, 74
 Mini Blueberry Pies, 139
 Mozzarella Bites, 116
 Open-Face Egg Sandwich, 33
 Parmesan Green Beans
  and Mushrooms, 105
 Peanut Butter Energy Bites, 112
 Pineapple Mojito Mocktail, 131

 Protein-Packed Strawberry
  Smoothie, 37
 Rainbow Fields Salad, 54
 Scrambled Egg Pita Pocket, 35
 Shredded Brussels Sprouts,
  Apples, and Pecans, 104
 Simple Coleslaw, 106
 Spinach Parmesan
  Spaghetti Squash, 89
 Strawberries and Cream, 133
 Tofu Stir-Fry, 94
 Traditional Caprese Salad, 117
 Veggie-Filled Omelet, 39
 Zucchini Bread, 148
Veggie-Filled Omelet, 39

W
Warm Lentil and Kale Soup, 59
Weight gain, 6, 8–9, 13
Wild Arugula, Spinach, and Steak
 Salad, 55

Y
Yogurt. *See also* Greek yogurt
 Broccoli Cream Soup, 62

Z
Zucchini
 Easy Black Bean Burger, 91
 Half Noodle Lasagna, 78
 Simple Veggie Soup, 66
 Zucchini Bread, 148

Symptoms Index

C

Constipation
Berry Parfait, 113
Butter Lettuce Salad
with Shrimp, 50
Citrus Snack Plate, 115
Easy Black Bean Burger, 91
Fresh Veggie Couscous, 109
Kale and Quinoa Salad, 51
Rainbow Fields Salad, 54
Roasted Broccoli with
Shallots, 102
Roasted Potatoes, Carrots,
and Asparagus, 101
Roasted Veggie Wrap, 82
Rustic Italian Salad, 52
Shredded Brussels Sprouts,
Apples, and Pecans, 104
Simple Coleslaw, 106
Taco Jar Salad, 53
Tofu Stir-Fry, 94
Veggie-Filled Omelet, 39
Warm Lentil and Kale Soup, 59
Wild Arugula, Spinach,
and Steak Salad, 55

E

Energy enhancers
Beef Stew, 96
Chicken and Wild Rice Soup, 61
Edamame Frittata, 42
Egg, Bacon, and Veggie
Breakfast Bake, 34
Kale and Quinoa Salad, 51
One-Pot Beef and Broccoli, 75
Open-Face Egg Sandwich, 33
Pan-Seared Rainbow Trout, 90
Peanut Butter Energy Bites, 112
Taco Jar Salad, 53
Two-Pan Turkey Dinner, 84
Veggie-Filled Omelet, 39

Wild Arugula, Spinach,
and Steak Salad, 55

G

Gestational diabetes-friendly
Almond-Crusted Cod, 81
Avocado Chicken Salad, 48
Baked Chicken Legs, 79
Cashew Chicken (or Tempeh)
Lettuce Wraps, 85
Cauliflower Mash, 108
Crave-Worthy Egg Salad, 46
Crustless Spinach Quiche, 43
Cumin Chicken and
Black Beans, 80
Egg, Bacon, and Veggie
Breakfast Bake, 34
Egg in Tomato Bake, 32
Home-Baked Kale Chips, 119
Kale and Quinoa Salad, 51
Lamb Kabobs, 88
Lemony Garlic Shrimp, 73
Mahi-Mahi Fish Tacos, 86
Mediterranean Roasted
Salmon, 92
Mozzarella Bites, 116
One-Pan Chicken and
Chickpea Bake, 72
Pan-Seared Rainbow Trout, 90
Parmesan Green Beans
and Mushrooms, 105
Pesto Chicken Salad, 49
Rainbow Chard–Stuffed
Chicken Breasts, 76
Roasted Broccoli with
Shallots, 102
Simple Go-To Salad
Dressing, 150
Simple Veggie Soup, 66
Spinach Parmesan
Spaghetti Squash, 89

Stuffed Avocado Salmon
Salad, 47
Sugar-Free Freshly Squeezed
Lemonade, 130
Traditional Caprese Salad, 117
Two-Pan Turkey Dinner, 84
Veggie-Filled Omelet, 39
Wild Arugula, Spinach,
and Steak Salad, 55

H

Headaches
Butter Lettuce Salad
with Shrimp, 50
Electrolyte Balance, 127
Kale and Quinoa Salad, 51
Kiwi, Cucumber, Kale
Smoothie, 40
Lemony Garlic Shrimp, 73
Mediterranean Roasted
Salmon, 92
Stuffed Avocado Salmon
Salad, 47

L

Lactation
Almond-Crusted Cod, 81
Carrot Cake for Breakfast, 29
Easy Black Bean Burger, 91
Lactation Cookies, 140
Lactation Tea Blend, 129
Pan-Seared Rainbow Trout, 90
Peanut Butter Energy Bites, 112
Rainbow Fields Salad, 54
Stuffed Avocado Salmon
Salad, 47
Sweet Potato Muffins, 41
Leg cramps
Avocado Chicken Salad, 48
Classic Tomato Soup and
Grilled Cheese, 57–58
Leg cramps (continued)

Delicata Squash Soup, 63–64
Easy Chicken Chili, 60
Electrolyte Balance, 127
Kiwi, Cucumber, Kale
      Smoothie, 40
One-Pot Beef and Broccoli, 75
Secret Ingredient Beef Chili, 67
Shredded Brussels Sprouts,
      Apples, and Pecans, 104
Spinach Parmesan
      Spaghetti Squash, 89
Stuffed Avocado Salmon
      Salad, 47
Sweet Potato Muffins, 41
Tofu Miso Soup, 68–69

N
Nausea
   Avocado Chicken Salad, 48
   Classic Tomato Soup and
         Grilled Cheese, 57–58
   Creamy Potato Soup, 65
   Easy Chicken Chili, 60
   Electrolyte Balance, 127
   Knockout Nausea Water, 125
   Mango Carrot Smoothie, 38
   Nausea-Diffusing Blend, 144
   Protein-Packed Strawberry
         Smoothie, 37
   Simple Veggie Soup, 66
   Sweet Potato Muffins, 41
   Zucchini Bread, 148

P
Postpartum recovery
   Beef Stew, 96
   Berry- and Basil-Infused
         Water, 126
   Broccoli Cream Soup, 62
   Cauliflower Mash, 108
   Cheesy Mini Quiches, 30
   Chicken and Wild Rice Soup, 61

Classic Tomato Soup and
      Grilled Cheese, 57–58
Creamy Potato Soup, 65
Delicata Squash Soup, 63–64
Easy Chicken Chili, 60
Edamame Frittata, 42
Egg, Bacon, and Veggie
      Breakfast Bake, 34
Half Noodle Lasagna, 78
Knockout Nausea Water, 125
Lactation Tea Blend, 129
Lentil and Quinoa
      "Meat"balls, 74
Mozzarella Bites, 116
One-Pan Chicken and
      Chickpea Bake, 72
One-Pot Beef and Broccoli, 75
Pesto Chicken Salad, 49
Relaxing Face Mask, 145
Roasted Chickpeas, 114
Sausage with Apple Sauerkraut
      and Potatoes, 95
Savory Meatballs with
      Egg Noodles, 97
Secret Ingredient Beef Chili, 67
Slow-Cooked Pulled Pork, 77
Spinach Parmesan
      Spaghetti Squash, 89
Stretch Mark Cream, 147
Sweet Potato Fries, 103
Three-Green Ancient Blend, 107
Tofu Miso Soup, 68–69
Turkey Arugula Pasta, 93
Warm Lentil and Kale Soup, 59
Pre-conception
   Artichoke, Spinach, and
         White Bean Dip, 120
   Baked Chicken Legs, 79
   Berry Parfait, 113
   Butter Lettuce Salad
         with Shrimp, 50
   Cheesy Mini Quiches, 30

Citrus Snack Plate, 115
Classic Deviled Eggs, 121
Crave-Worthy Egg Salad, 46
Create Your Own Flatbread, 83
Cumin Chicken and
      Black Beans, 80
Edamame Frittata, 42
Egg in Tomato Bake, 32
Fresh Veggie Couscous, 109
Kale and Quinoa Salad, 51
Lemony Garlic Shrimp, 73
Mango Carrot Smoothie, 38
Pesto Chicken Salad, 49
Rainbow Chard–Stuffed
      Chicken Breasts, 76
Roasted Potatoes, Carrots,
      and Asparagus, 101
Scrambled Egg Pita Pocket, 35
Taco Jar Salad, 53
Turmeric Hummus, 111
Two-Pan Turkey Dinner, 84
Warm Lentil and Kale Soup, 59
Wild Arugula, Spinach,
      and Steak Salad, 55

S
Swelling
   Avocado Chicken Salad, 48
   Avocado Chocolate
         Pudding, 138
   Berry- and Basil-Infused
         Water, 126
   Egg, Bacon, and Veggie
         Breakfast Bake, 34
   Egg in Tomato Bake, 32
   Electrolyte Balance, 127
   Rainbow Chard–Stuffed
         Chicken Breasts, 76
   Taco Jar Salad, 53

Acknowledgments

I would like to express my gratitude to everyone who has helped me get to the point in my career that's enabled me to write this book. I am truly blessed in so many ways to be surrounded by family, friends, coaches, professors, and mentors who believe in me and push me to be the best version of myself in my career and personal life. I would like to give an extra special thank-you to my mom, who became my sidekick in making this book what it is. Growing up, she taught me how to navigate the kitchen and, most importantly, how to create delicious and healthy food. I'm overwhelmed with joy at how this book has come together, and I look forward to what is to come.

About the Author

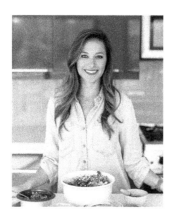

RYANN KIPPING is a clinically trained registered dietitian nutritionist (RDN) and certified lactation education counselor (CLEC). She is the founder of The Prenatal Nutritionist, a virtual nutrition private practice that focuses on preparing women for pregnancy and mastering nutrition during and after pregnancy. She helps women feel confident in their ability to properly nourish a growing baby through a real-food, holistic approach. With more than 200 documented hours of continuing education after passing the national exam to become a registered dietitian nutritionist, she makes it a top priority to stay up-to-date on the newest nutrition science and research. Aside from providing one-on-one nutrition counseling, Ryann is a nutrition writer, menu developer, and recipe creator. You can find her most often on her popular Instagram account @prenatalnutritionist.

CPSIA information can be obtained
at www.ICGtesting.com
Printed in the USA
BVHW051548280121
598616BV00004B/4